HUMAN RESOURCE DEVELOPMENT

HUMAN RESOURCE DEVELOPMENT

Dr. M.S. Talawar
M.A., M.Ed., Ph.d
Professor in Education &
Director-UGC-Academic Staff College
Central College Campus
Bangalore University
Bangalore-01, Karnataka

and

T. Pradeep Kumar
M.Ed., M.Phil, UGC-NET., PGDELT, PGDHE, PGDCA
Ph.d. Research Scholar
P.G. Department of Education
Bangalore University
Bangalore, Karnataka

A P H PUBLISHING CORPORATION
4435-36/7, ANSARI ROAD, DARYA GANJ
NEW DELHI-110 002

Published by
S.B. Nangia
A.P.H. Publishing Corporation
4435–36/7, Ansari Road, Darya Ganj,
New Delhi-110002
Phone: 011–23274050
e-mail: aphbooks@gmail.com

2026

Typeset by
Ideal Publishing Solutions
C-90, J.D. Cambridge School,
West Vinod Nagar, Delhi-110092

Printed at
DIVINE DIGITAL PRINTERS
Ansari road Daryaganj Delhi-110002

PREFACE

The **Ministry of Human Resource Development (HRD)** is an *Indian government ministry*, responsible for the development of *human resources*. The ministry is divided into two *departments*: the **Department of School Education and Literacy**, which deals with *primary education* and *literacy*, and the **Department of Higher Education**, which deals with *secondary* and *post-secondary education.*

Human Resource Development is a framework for the expansion of *human capital* within an organization. *Human Resources Development* is a combination of Training and Education that ensures the continual improvement and growth of both the individual and the organization. *Adam Smith* states, "The capacities of individuals depended on their access to education". (Kelly, 2001). The focus of all aspects of Human Resource Development is on developing the most superior workforce so that the organization and individual employees can accomplish their work goals in service to customers.

This book provides an Ever-broadening framework for the Human Resource Development in order to facilitate the readers in understanding the topics. It fulfills the needs and requirements in developing a prosperous society. Human Resources is a broader concept which covers a various information in this book. It meets the requirements of all the learners of Undergraduate and Post graduate irrespective of their education fields. Several sources both print and Electronic media have been also helpful for the writers of this book.

We express our gratitude to APH Publishing Corporation – **Sri Dr. K.B. NANGIA**, Managing Director. T. Pradeep Kumar Express heart felt thanks to family members – Father **J.V. Thimme Gowda**, Mother **Nagarathna**, Brother **T. Santhosh Kumar** - Software engineer, U.S.A,. **Keerthi** - Principal, ST. Mary's Institution, Vijayanagar, Bangalore, My Teachers and Mentors **Dr. M.S. Talawar, Dr. H.M. Kashinath, Dr. K.B. Praveen, Dr. G. Sheela** with whose support and co-operation this work was possible.

Dr. M.S. Talawar
T. Pradeep Kumar

CONTENTS

ABOUT THE AUTHOR

Dr. M.S. Talawar is presently working as a Professor in Education and Director –UGC-Academic Staff College, Bangalore University, Bangalore, Karnataka, India. He has 31 years of Teaching Experience in the field of Education.

He has published 14 books and 27 articles in the National Journals, presented 45 Thematic and Research Papers in National and International Conferences and has organized 14 different National level Programmes. Guided 100 M.Ed dissertation students, 22 M.phil. Students, 12 Ph.D. Scholars. He visited Philippines Under UGC Sponsored Cultural Exchange Programme to Undertake a Research on "A Comparative Study of Elementary Teacher Training Programme in India and Philippines", during 1997.

He has handled the post with prestigious Bodies like Chairman NAAC Peer Committee to Kambhat (Gujarat) and Member NAAC Peer Committee to Satara (Maharastra), Member Regional Committee to Central Board for Workers Education (Bangalore Unit) Ministry of Labour and Employment, Govt. of India, Member UGC Expert Committee to Review progress of X Plan and XI Plan proposal to Punjabi University, Patiala 2008, Member UGC Expert Committee to Review progress of X plan and XI plan proposal to Periyar University, Salem –25-27 Nov 2008. Expert Member of Visiting Committee NCTE SRC Bangalore.

ABOUT THE AUTHOR

T. Pradeep Kumar is Presently Research Scholar in the Post Graduate Department of Education, Bangalore University, Bangalore, Karnataka, India. Formerly Lecturer in P.E.T College of Education, Bangalore, Karnataka. He got Educational Qualifications such as M.Ed., M.Phil, UGC-NET, PGDELT, PGDHE, PGDCA. He was awarded 4th Rank in M.Ed.; Bangalore University in the year 2005-06.

He has Published 3 Books and 5 Articles in the National Journals. Presented 15 Thematic and Research Papers in National and International Conferences. His Research areas of Interest are Educational Technology, Educational Psychology, Teacher Absenteeism, and Academic Achievement.

ABOUT THE BOOK

The **Ministry of Human Resource Development (HRD)** is an Indian government ministry, responsible for the development of human resources. The ministry is divided into two departments: the **Department of School Education and Literacy**, which deals with primary education and literacy, and the **Department of Higher Education**, which deals with secondary and post-secondary education.

Human Resource Development is the framework for helping employees develops their personal and organizational skills, knowledge, and abilities. Human Resource Development includes such opportunities as employee training, employee career development, performance management and development, coaching, succession planning, key employee identification, tuition assistance, and organization development.

The focus of all aspects of Human Resource Development is on developing the most superior workforce so that the organization and individual employees can accomplish their work goals in service to customers. Human Resource Development can be formal such as in classroom training, a college course, or an organizational planned change effort. Or, Human Resource Development can be informal as in employee coaching by a manager. Healthy organizations believe in Human Resource Development and cover all of these bases.

This book is prepared keeping in mind of all the aspects required in improving the process and product of Human Resource Development which is confronting the essential needs and requirements for development of Society through various fields like Education, Management, Organizations, Planning, Training, Industrial fields, Economy etc. It meets the requirements of all the learners of Undergraduate and Post graduate irrespective of their education fields.

There are nine units in this Book which covers broad concepts like Introduction to HRD, Ministry of HRD in India, Human Resource Management, Concept of Human Resource system, Human

Resource Planning, Functional Planning, Human Resource Development Mechanisms, Analysis, Reward Management, Training in HRD, HRD and Organization effectiveness, HRD Climate, Performance appraisal, Psychological strategies of HRD, Organizational Development in HRD, HRD Committee, HRD for Women, HRD and Small scale sector, HRD and functional literacy, Models in HRD, Behavioral model in HRD, Career Development in HRD, Integrated HRD Systems, HRD and Management, Barriers to HRD, HRD and Social Change, Research and Development in HRD, HRD Approaches, Professionalization in HRD, Problems and issues din HRD, HRD Evaluation, Counselling in HRD, Job enrichment, Quality of working life, HRD linkages.

UNIT 1

INTRODUCTION TO HUMAN RESOURCE DEVELOPMENT

Human Resource Development is the framework for helping employees develops their personal and organizational skills, knowledge, and abilities. Human Resource Development includes such opportunities as employee training, employee career development, performance management and development, coaching, succession planning, key employee identification, tuition assistance, and organization development.

The focus of all aspects of Human Resource Development is on developing the most superior workforce so that the organization and individual employees can accomplish their work goals in service to customers.

Human Resource Development can be formal such as in classroom training, a college course, or an organizational planned change effort. Or, Human Resource Development can be informal as in employee coaching by a manager. Healthy organizations believe in Human Resource Development and cover all of these bases.

Human Resources Development is a framework for the expansion of *human capital* within an organization. *Human Resources Development* is a combination of Training and Education that ensures the continual improvement and growth of both the individual and the organization. *Adam Smith* states, "The capacities of individuals depended on their access to education". (Kelly, 2001).

Human Resources Development is the medium that drives the process between training and learning. Human Resources Development is not a defined object, but a series of organised processes, "with a specific learning objective" (Nadler, 1984) Human

Resources Development is the structure that allows for individual development, potentially satisfying the organisation's goals. The development of the individual will benefit both the individual and the organisation. The Human Resources Development framework views employees, as an asset to the enterprise whose value will be enhanced by development, "Its primary focus is on growth and employee development it emphasises developing individual potential and skills" (Elwood, Holton and Trott 1996) Human Resources Development can be in-room group training, tertiary or vocational courses or mentoring and coaching by senior employees with the aim for a desired outcome that will develop the individual's performance. An apprentice will step through the development process to become a tradesman in their field as will a white-collar trainee to become a professional in their field. Training will allow the individual to complete a task within their field today Gutteridge and Hutcheson maintain that, "Training provides, maintains and enhances skills to perform the job" (Nadler 1984) Education and training will develop the individual to become a tradesman or a professional in the future. A successful Human Resources Development program will prepare the individual to undertake a higher level of work, "organised learning over a given period of time, to provide the possibility of performance change" (Nadler 1984). Human Resources Development is the framework that focuses on the organisations competencies at the first stage, training, and then developing the employee, through education, to satisfy the organisations long-term needs and the individuals' career goals and employee value to their present and future employers. Human Resources Development can be defined simply as developing the most important section of any business its human resource by, "attaining or upgrading the skills and attitudes of employees at all levels in order to maximise the effectiveness of the enterprise" (Kelly 2001). The people within an organization are its human resource. Human Resources Development from a business perspective is not entirely focused on the individual's growth and development, "development occurs to enhance the organization's value, not solely for individual improvement. Individual education and development is a tool and a means to an end, not the end goal itself". (Elwood F. Holton II, James W. Trott Jr.).

In organizations, in terms of selection it is important to consider carrying out a thorough *job analysis* to determine the level of skills/technical abilities, competencies, flexibility of the employee required etc. At this point it is important to consider both the internal and external factors that can have an effect on the recruitment of employees. The external factors are those out-with the powers of the organization and include issues such as current and future trends of the labor market e.g. skills, education level, government investment into industries etc. On the other hand internal influences are easier to control, predict and monitor, for example management *styles* or even the *organizational culture.*

MAJOR TRENDS

In order to know the business environment in which any organization operates, three major trends should be considered:

- *Demographics* – the characteristics of a population/workforce, for example, age, gender or social class. This type of trend may have an effect in relation to pension offerings, insurance packages etc.
- *Diversity* – the variation within the population/workplace. Changes in society now mean that a larger proportion of organizations are made up of "*baby-boomers*" or older employees in comparison to thirty years ago. Traditional advocates of "workplace diversity" simply advocate an employee base that is a mirror reflection of the make-up of society insofar as race, gender, sexual orientation, etc.
- **Skills and qualifications** – as industries move from manual to more managerial professions so does the need for more highly skilled graduates. If the market is "tight" (i.e. not enough staff for the jobs), employers will have to compete for employees by offering financial rewards, community investment, etc.

INDIVIDUAL RESPONSES

In regard to how individuals respond to the changes in a labour market the following should be understood:

- **Geographical spread** – how far is the job from the individual? The distance to travel to work should be in line with the pay offered by the organization and the transportation and infrastructure of the area will also be an influencing factor in deciding who will apply for a post.

- **Occupational structure** – the norms and values of the different careers within an organization. Mahoney 1989 developed 3 different types of occupational structure namely craft (loyalty to the profession), organization career (promotion through the firm) and unstructured (lower/unskilled workers who work when needed).
- **Generational difference** – different age categories of employees have certain characteristics, for example their behavior and their expectations of the organization.

RECRUITMENT METHODS

While recruitment methods are wide and varied, it is important that the job is described correctly and that any personal specifications are stated. Job recruitment methods can be through job centres, employment agencies/consultants, headhunting, and local/national newspapers. It is important that the correct media is chosen to ensure an appropriate response to the advertised post.

Where organisations don't have the internal resource to be able to conduct an effective recruitment exercise this is where they may outsource this to a third party, typically a recruitment or consultancy that specialises in the area that the organisation requires.

FRAMEWORK

Human Resources Development is a framework for the expansion of human capital within an organization or (in new approaches) a municipality, region, or nation. Human Resources Development is a combination of training and education, in a broad context of adequate health and employment policies, that ensures the continual improvement and growth of both the individual, the organisation, and the national human resourcefulness. Adam Smith states, "The capacities of individuals depended on their access to education". Human Resources Development is the medium that drives the process between training and learning in a broadly fostering environment. Human Resources Development is not a defined object, but a series of organised processes, "with a specific learning objective" (Nadler, 1984) Within a national context, it becomes a strategic approach to intersectoral linkages between health, education and employment.

STRUCTURE

Human Resources Development is the structure that allows for individual development, potentially satisfying the organization's, or the nation's goals. The development of the individual will benefit both the individual, the organization, or the nation and its citizens. In the corporate vision, the Human Resources Development framework views employees, as an asset to the enterprise whose value will be enhanced by development, "Its primary focus is on growth and employee development... i.e. emphasises developing individual potential and skills" (Elwood, Olton and Trott 1996) Human Resources Development in this treatment can be in-room group training, tertiary or vocational courses or mentoring and coaching by senior employees with the aim for a desired outcome that will develop the individual's performance. At the level of a national strategy, it can be a broad intersectoral approach to fostering creative contributions to national productivity.

TRAINING

At the organizational level, a successful Human Resources Development program will prepare the individual to undertake a higher level of work, "organized learning over a given period of time, to provide the possibility of performance change" (Nadler 1984). In these settings, Human Resources Development is the framework that focuses on the organizations competencies at the first stage, training, and then developing the employee, through education, to satisfy the organizations long-term needs and the individuals' career goals and employee value to their present and future employers. Human Resources Development can be defined simply as developing the most important section of any business its human resource by, "attaining or upgrading the skills and attitudes of employees at all levels in order to maximise the effectiveness of the enterprise" (Kelly 2001). The people within an organization are its human resource. Human Resources Development from a business perspective is not entirely focused on the individual's growth and development, "development occurs to enhance the organization's value, not solely for individual improvement. Individual education and development is a tool and a means to an end, not the end goal itself". (Elwood F. Holton II, James W. Trott Jr) The broader concept of national and more strategic attention to the development of human resources is beginning to emerge as newly independent countries face strong competition for their skilled professionals and the accompanying brain-drain they experience.

MODERN CONCEPT OF HUMAN RESOURCES

Though human resources have been part of business and organizations since the first days of agriculture, the modern concept of human resources began in reaction to the efficiency focus of *Taylorism* in the early 1900s. By 1920, psychologists and employment experts in the *United States* started the *human relations* movement, which viewed workers in terms of their *psychology* and fit with companies, rather than as interchangeable parts. This movement grew throughout the middle of the 20th century, placing emphasis on how *leadership*, cohesion, and loyalty played important roles in organizational success. Although this view was increasingly challenged by more quantitatively rigorous and less "soft" management techniques in the 1960s and beyond, human resources development had gained a permanent role within organizations, agencies and nations, increasingly as not only an academic discipline, but as a central theme in development policy.

MINISTRY OF HUMAN RESOURCE DEVELOPMENT (INDIA)

The **Ministry of Human Resource Development (HRD)** is an *Indian government ministry*, responsibie for the development of *human resources*. The ministry is divided into two *departments*: the **Department of School Education and Literacy**, which deals with *primary education* and *literacy*, and the **Department of Higher Education**, which deals with *secondary* and *post-secondary education*.

The Ministry of Human Resource Development is headed by a minister of *cabinet* rank as a member of the *Council of Ministers*.

The current Minister of Human Resource Development is *Kapil Sibal*. The minister is assisted by two *Ministers of State*, one for each department: *Ali Ashraf Fatmi* (Minister of State for School Education and Literacy) and *Daggubati Purandeswari* (Minister of State for Higher Education).

DEPARTMENT OF SCHOOL EDUCATION AND LITERACY

The Department of School Education and Literacy is responsible for primary education, both formal and non-formal. Its stated goal is the universalization of elementary education (UEE). The department originated as the Indian Education Department in the 1910 under the *British Raj*. After *independence*, a full-fledged ministry, the **Ministry of Education**, was created in 1947. The Ministry of Education was merged with the newly-created Ministry of Human Resource Development in 1985. The department aims to achieve universal access and *enrollment*, universal retention of children up to 14 years of age, and substantial improvement in the quality of education to enable all children to achieve essential levels of learning.

DEPARTMENT OF HIGHER EDUCATION

The Department of Higher Education is in charge of secondary and post-secondary education.

The Department is divided into six *bureaus*: University and Higher Education; Minorities Education; Book Promotion and Copyrights; Technical Education; Distance Education and Scholarships; Planning; and UNESCO, International Cooperation, Administration, Coordination, Policy, Statistics, and Languages; and the Integrated Finance Division.

Most the work of the department is through about 90 autonomous bodies that it oversees are:

- *University Grants Commission* (UGC), the 23 *Central Universities* (Union Universities), the *Indian Council of Social Science Research* (ICSSR), the *Indian Council of Historical Research* (ICHR), the *Indian Council of Philosophical Research* (ICPR), and the *Indian Institute of Advanced Studies* (IIAS), *Shimla*.

- *All India Council for Technical Education* (AICTE), the seven *Indian Institutes of Technology* (IITs), the three *Indian Institutes of Science Education and Research* (IISERs), the six *Indian Institutes of Management* (IIMs), the 20 *National Institutes of Technology* (NITs), the four *Indian Institutes of Information Technology* (IIITs), the four *National Institutes of Technical Teachers' Training and Research* (NITTTRs), and the four Regional Boards of Apprenticeship/Practical Training
- The three Deemed Universities in the field of *Sanskrit* [*Rashtriya Sanskrit Sansthan* (RSkS)], New Delhi; *Shri Lal Bahadur Shastri Rashtriya Sanskrit Vidyapeeth* (SLBSRSV), New Delhi; and *Rashtriya Sanskrit Vidyapeeth* (RSV), Tirupati), *Kendriya Hindi Sansthan* (KHS), *Agra*; the *Central Institute of English and Foreign Languages* (CIEFL), *Hyderabad*; the *National Council for Promotion of Urdu Language* (NCPUL); and *National Council for Promotion of Sindhi Language* (NCPSL)
- *National Institute of Educational Planning and Administration* (NIEPA)
- *National Book Trust* (NBT)
- *National Commission for Minority Educational Institutions* (NCMEI)
- Attached Offices: Central Hindi Directorate, New Delhi; Commission for Scientific and Technical Terminology (CSTT), New Delhi; Central Institute of Indian Languages (CIL), Mysore
- A *public sector enterprise*, *Educational Consultants (India) Limited* (EdCIL)
- *National Council of Educational Research and Training* (NCERT)
- *Central Board of Secondary Education* (CBSE)
- *Kendriya Vidyalaya Sangathan* (KVS)
- *Navodaya Vidyalaya Samiti* (NVS)
- *National Institute of Open Schooling* (NIOS)
- *Central Tibetan School Administration* (CTSA)
- *National Foundation for Teachers' Welfare*

And the following post-secondary education bodies are:

- *University Grants Commission* (UGC) - responsible for coordination, determination and maintenance of standards, release of grants.
- Professional councils, responsible for recognition of courses, promotion of professional institutions and providing grants to undergraduate programmes and various awards:
  - *All India Council for Technical Education* (AICTE)
  - *Distance Education Council* (DEC)
  - *Indian Council for Agriculture Research* (ICAR)
  - *Bar Council of India* (BCI)
  - *National Council for Teacher Education* (NCTE)
  - *Rehabilitation Council of India* (RCI)
  - *Medical Council of India* (MCI)
  - Pharmacy Council of India (PCI)
  - Indian Nursing Council (INC)
  - Dentist Council of India (DCI)
  - Central Council of Homeopathy (CCH)
  - Central Council of Indian Medicine (CCIM)

As well as following *Inter University Centres* (IUCs) are:

- *Nuclear Science Centre*, New Delhi
- *Inter University Centre for Astronomy and Astrophysics* (IUCAA), Pune
- *Inter University Consortium for DAE Facilities*, Indore
- *Information and Library Network* (INFLIBNET), Ahmedabad
- *Consortium for Educational Communication* (CEC)
- *National Assessment and Accreditation Council* (NACC), Bangalore

HUMAN RESOURCES

Human resources is an increasingly broadening term with which an organization, or other human system describes the combination of traditionally administrative personnel functions with acquisition and application of skills, knowledge and experience, Employee Relations and *resource* planning at various levels. The field draws upon concepts developed in Industrial/Organizational Psychology and *System Theory*. Human resources has at least two related interpretations depending on context. The original usage derives from *political economy* and *economics*, where it was traditionally called *labor*, one of four *factors of production* although this perspective is changing as a function of new and ongoing research into more strategic approaches at national levels. This first usage is used more in terms of 'human resources development', and can go beyond just organizations to the level of nations. The more traditional usage within corporations and businesses refers to the individuals within a firm or agency, and to the portion of the organization that deals with hiring, firing, training, and other personnel issues, typically referred to as 'human resources management'.

Development

The objective of human resource's' development (the 's' is important in human resource's' in that it underscores individuality/variability) is to foster human resourcefulness through enlightened and cohesive policies in education, training, health and employment at all levels, from corporate to national (Lawrence 2000).

Management

Human resource management's objective, on the other hand, is to maximize the return on investment from the organization's human capital and minimize financial risk. It is the responsibility of human resource managers in a corporate context to conduct these activities in an effective, legal, fair, and consistent manner.

Key functions

Human resource management serves these key functions:

1. Recruitment & Selection
2. Training and Development (People or Organization)
3. Performance Evaluation and Management
4. Promotions
5. Redundancy

6. Industrial and Employee Relations
7. Record keeping of all personal data
8. Compensation, pensions, bonuses etc. in liaison with Payroll
9. Confidential advice to internal 'customers' in relation to problems at work
10. Career development
11. Employee grievance redressal
12. Provides motivation
13. Job rotation

Modern analysis

Modern analysis emphasizes that human beings are not "*commodities*" or "resources", but are creative and social beings in a productive enterprise. The 2000 revision of *ISO 9001* in contrast requires to identify the processes, their sequence and interaction, and to define and communicate responsibilities and authorities. In general, heavily unionized nations such as *France* and *Germany* have adopted and encouraged such job descriptions especially within trade unions. The International Labour Organization also in 2001 decided to revisit, and revise its 1975 Recommendation 150 on Human Resources Development. One view of these trends is that a strong social consensus on political economy and a good *social welfare system* facilitates *labor mobility* and tends to make the entire economy more productive, as labor can develop skills and experience in various ways, and move from one enterprise to another with little controversy or difficulty in adapting. Another view is that governments should become more aware of their national role in facilitating human resources development across all sectors.

Controversy

Labour mobility

An important controversy regarding labor mobility illustrates the broader philosophical issue with usage of the phrase "human resources": governments of developing nations often regard developed nations that encourage immigration or "guest workers" as appropriating human capital that is rightfully part of the developing nation and required to further its growth as a *civilization*. They argue that this appropriation is similar to *colonial commodity fiat* wherein a colonizing European power would define an arbitrary price for *natural resources*, extracting which diminished national *natural capital*.

The debate regarding "human resources" versus human capital thus in many ways echoes the debate regarding natural resources versus natural capital. Over time the *United Nations* have come to more generally support the developing nations' point of view, and have requested significant offsetting "foreign aid" contributions so that a developing nation losing human capital does not lose the capacity to continue to train new people in trades, professions, and the arts.

An extreme version of this view is that historical inequities such as *African slavery* must be compensated by current developed nations, which benefited from stolen "human resources" as they were developing. This is an extremely controversial view, but it echoes the general theme of converting human capital to "human resources" and thus greatly diminishing its value to the host society, i.e. "Africa", as it is put to narrow imitative use as "labor" in the using society.

In a series of reports of the UN Secretary-General to the General Assembly [e.g. A/56/162 (2001)], a broad inter-sectoral approach to developing human resourcefulness [see United Nations Expert Meeting on Human Resources Development. Changing Perspectives on Human Resources Development. ST/TCD/SER.E/ 25. June 1994] has been outlined as a priority for socio-economic development and particularly anti-poverty strategies. This calls for strategic and integrated public policies, for example in education, health, and employment sectors that promote occupational skills, knowledge and performance enhancement (*Lawrence, J.E.S.*)

Perceptions

Terms like "human resources" and "human capital" may be perceived as insulting to people. They create the impression that people are merely commodities, like office machines or vehicles, despite assurances to the contrary.

Corporate management

In the very narrow context of corporate "human resources" management, there is a contrasting pull to reflect and require *workplace diversity* that echoes the diversity of a global customer base. Foreign language and culture skills, ingenuity, humor, and careful listening, are examples of traits that such programs typically require. It would appear that these evidence a general shift through the human capital point of view to an acknowledgment that human beings do contribute much more to a productive enterprise than "work": they bring their character, their ethics, their creativity, their social connections, and in some cases even their pets and children, and alter the character of a workplace. The term *corporate culture* is used to characterize such processes at the organizational level.

The traditional but extremely narrow context of hiring, firing, and job description is considered a 20th century anachronism. Most corporate organizations that compete in the modern global economy have adopted a view of human capital that mirrors the modern consensus as above. Some of these, in turn, deprecate the term "human resources" as useless. Yet the term survives, and if related to 'resourcefulness', has continued and emerging relevance to public policy.

In general the abstractions of macro-economics treat it this way - as it characterizes no mechanisms to represent choice or ingenuity. So one interpretation is that "firm-specific human capital" as defined in macro-economics is the modern and correct definition of "human resources" - and that this is inadequate to represent the contributions of "human resources" in any modern theory of *political economy*.

Training and development

In the field of *human resource management*, **training and development** is the field concerned with organizational activity aimed at bettering the performance of individuals and groups in organizational settings. It has been known by several names, including **employee development, human resource development**, and **learning and development**.

Harrison observes that the name was endlessly debated by the *Chartered Institute of Personnel and Development* during its review of professional standards in 1999/2000. "Employee Development" was seen as too evocative of the master-slave relationship between employer and employee for those who refer to their employees as "partners" or "associates" to be comfortable with. "Human Resource Development" was rejected by academics, who objected to the idea that people were "resources" — an idea that they felt to be demeaning to the individual. Eventually, the CIPD settled upon "Learning and Development", although that was itself not free from problems, "learning" being an over general and ambiguous name. Moreover, the field is still widely known by the other names.

Training and development encompasses three main activities: training, education, and development. Garavan, Costine, and Heraty, of the Irish Institute of Training and Development, note that these ideas are often considered to be synonymous. However, to practitioners, they encompass three separate, although interrelated, activities:

- **Training**

  This activity is both focused upon, and evaluated against, the job that an individual currently holds.
- **Education**

  This activity focuses upon the jobs that an individual may potentially hold in the future, and is evaluated against those jobs.
- **Development**

  This activity focuses upon the activities that the organization employing the individual, or that the individual is part of, may partake in the future, and is almost impossible to evaluate.

The "stakeholders" in training and development are categorized into several classes. The *sponsors* of training and development are senior managers. The *clients* of training and development are business planners. Line managers are responsible for coaching, resources, and performance. The *participants* are those who actually undergo the processes. The *facilitators* are Human Resource Management staff. And the *providers* are specialists in the field.

Each of these groups has its own agenda and motivations, which sometimes conflict with the agendas and motivations of the others.

The conflicts are the best part of career consequences are those that take place between employees and their bosses. The number one reason people leave their jobs is conflict with their bosses. And yet, as author, workplace relationship authority, and executive coach, Dr. John Hoover points out, "Tempting as it is, nobody ever enhanced his or her career by making the boss look stupid." Training an employee to get along well with authority and with people who entertain diverse points of view is one of the best guarantees of long-term success. Talent, knowledge, and skill alone won't compensate for a sour relationship with a superior, peer, or customer.

HUMAN RESOURCE MANAGEMENT

Introduction

The shift from orthodox personnel management to HRM is explained in terms of global economic developments. The 'first wave' critiques of HRM, represented by John Storey's seminal book, *New Perspectives on Human Resource Management* (1989), introduces students to the debate on the many contradictions associated with the HRM model. The 'second wave' critiques focus on outcomes, restructured organizational forms and relationships. Recent events have exposed traditional underlying tensions and paradoxes in managing the employment relationship.

The history of human resource management

The development of personnel management is linked to post-Second World War government economic policies (Keynesianism) and the introduction of employment law, government intervention in the workplace (for example training), recommendations of the Donovan Commission, and the growth of workplace trade unionism all account for the evolution of personnel management.

The HRM phenomenon is explained in terms of the renaissance of 'market disciplines' and the challenge to government intervention in the economy.

Human resource management (HRM) is the *strategic* and *coherent* approach to the *management* of an organisation's most valued assets - the people working there who individually and collectively contribute to the achievement of the objectives of the business. The terms "human resource management" and "human resources" (HR) have largely replaced the term "personnel management" as a description of the processes involved in managing people in organizations. In simple sense, HRM means employing people, developing their resources, utilizing, maintaining and compensating their services in tune with the job and organizational requirement.

Human resource management functions

To explore HRM functions the text addresses three questions: What do HR professionals do? What affects what they do? And how do HR professionals do what they do? We identify eight key HRM functions to answer the first question, including planning, staffing, developing, motivating, maintaining, managing relationships, managing change and evaluating.

We can identify three broad contingencies: external context, strategy and organizational design to address the question 'What affects what HR professionals do?' And a range of technical, cognitive and interpersonal processes and skills are used to accomplish HR functions.

Features

Its features include:

- Organizational management
- Personnel administration
- Manpower management
- Industrial management

But these traditional expressions are becoming less common for the theoretical discipline. Sometimes even *industrial relations* and employee relations are confusingly listed as synonyms, although these normally refer to the relationship between management and workers and the behavior of workers in companies.

The theoretical discipline is based primarily on the assumption that employees are individuals with varying goals and needs, and as such should not be thought of as basic business resources, such as trucks and filing cabinets. The field takes a positive view of workers, assuming that virtually all wish to contribute to the enterprise productively, and that the main obstacles to their endeavors are lack of knowledge, insufficient training, and failures of process.

HRM is seen by practitioners in the field as a more innovative view of workplace management than the traditional approach. Its techniques force the managers of an enterprise to express their goals with specificity so that they can be understood and undertaken by the workforce, and to provide the resources needed for them to successfully accomplish their assignments. As such, HRM techniques, when properly practiced, are expressive of the goals and operating practices of the enterprise overall. HRM is also seen by many to have a key role in risk reduction within organizations.

Synonyms such as *personnel management* are often used in a more restricted sense to describe activities that are necessary in the recruiting of a workforce, providing its members with payroll and benefits, and administrating their work-life needs. So if we move to actual definitions, Torrington and Hall (1987) define personnel management as being:

"a series of activities which: first enable working people and their employing organisations to agree about the objectives and nature of their working relationship and, secondly, ensures that the agreement is fulfilled" (p. 49).

While Miller (1987) suggests that HRM relates to:

".......those decisions and actions which concern the management of employees at all levels in the business and which are related to the implementation of strategies directed towards creating and sustaining competitive advantage" (p. 352).

Theoretical perspectives on HRM

It is evident from reviewing the literature that the meaning and theoretical significance of HRM is contested. The controversy centres on at least two fundamental questions: (1) what exactly does

HRM mean and how, if at all, does it differ from personnel management? (2) What core values underlie the HRM model?

The five theoretical models of HRM

a. Fombrun, Tichy and Devanna model of HRM
b. Harvard model of HRM
c. Guest model of HRM
d. Warwick model of HRM
e. Storey model of HRM

HRM models emphasize a number of differences between the 'new' HRM and traditional personnel management. These include: strategic planning, focus on the psychological contract, importance of learning in the workplace, focus on the individual (unitarism), importance of leadership and proactive ness, a focus on line managers and an attention to measuring HR performance outcomes.

The critiques of HRM focus on the internal paradoxes and tensions, including the HR role of caring and controlling, the 'soft' and 'hard' schools of HRM, leaders gaining control by giving it up, short-term accounting practices versus long-term HR developmental practices, and the tendency for the HRM discourse to be 'gender-blind'.

Studying human resource management

The analysis of HRM needs to appreciate how the discipline is divided into theoretical traditions or strands of thought. The two strands of thought or 'standpoints' we come across are mainstream managerial and critical. The theoretical roots of the managerial standpoint can be traced back to the work of F.W. Taylor. The theoretical roots of the critical standpoint can be traced back to the radical sociological analysis of work and industry by Karl Marx.

Academic theory

The goal of human resource management is to help an organization to meet strategic goals by attracting, and maintaining employees and also to manage them effectively. The key word here perhaps is "fit", i.e. a HRM approach seeks to ensure a fit between the management of an organization's employees, and the overall strategic direction of the company (Miller, 1989).

The basic premise of the academic theory of HRM is that humans are not machines, therefore we need to have an interdisciplinary examination of people in the workplace. Fields such as *psychology*, industrial engineering, industrial, Legal/Paralegal Studies and organizational psychology, industrial relations, *sociology*, and critical theories: *postmodernism, post-structuralism* play a major role. Many colleges and universities offer bachelor and master degrees in Human Resources Management.

One widely used scheme to describe the role of HRM, developed by *Dave Ulrich*, defines 4 fields for the HRM function:

- Strategic business partner
- *Change management*
- Employee champion
- Administration

However, many HR functions these days struggle to get beyond the roles of administration and employee champion, and are seen rather as reactive than strategically proactive partners for the top management. In addition, HR organizations also have the difficulty in proving how their activities and processes add value to the company. Only in the recent years HR scholars and HR professionals are focusing to develop models that can measure if HR adds value.

Critical Academic Theory

Postmodernism plays an important part in Academic Theory and particularly in Critical Theory. Indeed Karen Legge in 'Human Resource Management: Rhetorics and Realities' poses the debate of whether HRM is a modernist project or a postmodern discourse (Legge 2004). In many ways, critically or not, many writers contend that HRM itself is an attempt to move away from the modernist traditions of personnel (man as machine) towards a postmodernist view of HRM (man as individuals). Critiques include the notion that because 'Human' is the subject we should recognize that people are complex and that it is only through various discourses that we understand the world. Man is not Machine, no matter what attempts are made to change it i.e. *Fordism/Taylorism, McDonaldisation* (Modernism).

Critical Theory also questions whether HRM is the pursuit of "attitudinal shaping" (Wilkinson 1998), particularly when considering empowerment, or perhaps more precisely pseudo-empowerment - as the critical perspective notes. Many critics note the move away from Man as Machine is often in many ways, more a Linguistic (discursive) move away than a real attempt to recognize the Human in Human Resource Management.

Critical Theory, in particular postmodernism (post-structuralism), recognizes that because the subject is people in the workplace, the subject is a complex one, and therefore simplistic notions of 'the best way' or unitary perspectives on the subject are too simplistic. It also considers the complex subject of *power*, power games, and *office politics*. Power in the workplace is a vast and complex subject that cannot be easily defined. This leaves many critics to suggest that Management 'Gurus', consultants, 'best practice' and HR models are often overly simplistic, but in order to sell an idea, they are simplified, and often lead Management as a whole to fall into the trap of oversimplifying the relationship.

Business practice

Human resources management comprises several processes. Together they are supposed to achieve the above mentioned goal. These processes can be performed in an HR department, but some tasks can also be outsourced or performed by line-managers or other departments. When effectively integrated they provide significant economic benefit to the company. .

- *Workforce planning*
- *Recruitment* (sometimes separated into attraction and selection)
- *Induction* and *Orientation*
- *Skills management*
- *Training and development*
- Personnel administration
- Compensation in *wage* or *salary*
- *Time management*
- Travel management (sometimes assigned to accounting rather than HRM)

- *Payroll* (sometimes assigned to accounting rather than HRM)
- *Employee benefits* administration
- Personnel cost planning
- Performance Appraisal

Careers

The sort of careers available in HRM are varied. There are generalist HRM jobs such as human resource assistant. There are careers involved with employment, recruitment and placement and these are usually conducted by interviewers, EEO (*Equal Employment Opportunity*) specialists or college recruiters. Training and development specialism is often conducted by trainers and orientation specialists. Compensation and benefits tasks are handled by compensation analysts, salary administrators, and benefits administrators.

Professional organizations

Professional organizations in HRM include the *Society for Human Resource Management*, the Australian Human Resources Institute (AHRI), the *Chartered Institute of Personnel and Development* (CIPD), the International Public Management Association for HR (IPMA-HR), Management Association of Nepal *MAN* and the International Personnel Management Association of Canada (IPMA-Canada), Human Capital Institute (HCI).

Functions

The Human Resources Management (HRM) function includes a variety of activities, and key among them is deciding what staffing needs you have and whether to use independent contractors or hire employees to fill these needs, recruiting and training the best employees, ensuring they are high performers, dealing with performance issues, and ensuring your personnel and management practices conform to various regulations. Activities also include managing your approach to employee benefits and compensation, employee records and personnel policies. Usually small businesses (for-profit or nonprofit) have to carry out these activities themselves because they can't yet afford part- or full-time help. However, they should always ensure that employees have – and are aware of –

personnel policies which conform to current regulations. These policies are often in the form of employee manuals, which all employees have.

Note that some people distinguish a difference between between HRM (a major management activity) and HRD (Human Resource Development, a profession). Those people might include HRM in HRD, explaining that HRD includes the broader range of activities to develop personnel inside of organizations, including, e.g., career development, training, organization development, etc.

There is a long-standing argument about where HR-related functions should be organized into large organizations, e.g., "should HR be in the Organization Development department or the other way around?"

The HRM· function and HRD profession have undergone tremendous change over the past 20-30 years. Many years ago, large organizations looked to the "Personnel Department," mostly to manage the paperwork around hiring and paying people. More recently, organizations consider the "HR Department" as playing a major role in staffing, training and helping to manage people so that people and the organization are performing at maximum capability in a highly fulfilling manner.

CHANGING NATURE OF HUMAN RESOURCE MANAGEMENT

HR Management Challenges

The environment faced by HR management is a challenging one; changes are occurring rapidly across a wide range of issues. A study by the Hudson Institute, entitled *Workforce 2020,* has highlighted some of the most important workforce issues. From that and other sources, it appears that the most prevalent challenges facing HR management are as follows:

- Economic and technological change
- Workforce availability and quality concerns
- Demographics and diversity issues
- Organizational restructuring

Economic and Technological Change

Several economic changes have occurred that have altered employment and occupational Patterns. A major change is the shift of jobs from manufacturing and agriculture to service industries and telecommunications. This shift has meant that some organizations have had to reduce the number of employees, while others have had to attract and retain employees with different capabilities than previously were needed. Additionally, pressures from global competitors have forced many firms to close facilities, adapt their management practices, and increase productivity and decrease labor costs in order to become more competitive. Finally, the explosive growth of information technology particularly that linked to the Internet has forced many changes throughout organizations of all types.

OCCUPATIONAL SHIFTS

A projection of the growth and decline in jobs illustrates the economic and employment shifts currently occurring. The occupations with the largest percentage growth anticipated between 1996 and 2006. It is interesting to note that most of the fastest-growing occupations percentages wise are related to information technology or health care. The increase in the technology jobs is due to the rapid increase in the use of information technology, such as databases, system design and analysis, and desktop publishing.

Human Resource (HR) management

The design of formal systems in an organization to ensure the effective and efficient use of human talent to accomplish the organizational goals.

GLOBAL COMPETITION

One major factor affecting these shifts is the globalization of economic forces. As seen the past few years, the collapse of Asian economies had significant effects on organizations. This is particularly true with more highly skilled, technical jobs in technology-driven industries. On the other hand, the less-skilled manufacturing assembly jobs have been shifting from the higher-wage, Due to the increase in information technology, global linkages are now more extensive and production and transportation can be coordinated worldwide. Therefore the loss of manufacturing jobs has been replaced with jobs in information technology.

WORKFORCE QUALITY DEFICIT

Many occupational groups and industries will require more educated workers in the coming years. The number of jobs requiring advanced knowledge is expected to grow at a much more rapid rate than the number of other jobs. This growth means that people without high school diplomas or appropriate college degrees increasingly will be at a disadvantage, as their Employment opportunities are confined to the lowest-paying service jobs. In short, there is a growing gap between the knowledge and skills required by many jobs and those possessed by employees and applicants. Several different studies and projections all point to the likelihood that employers in many industries will have difficulties obtaining sufficiently educated and trained workers.

Unless major efforts are made to improve educational systems, especially those serving minorities, employers will be unable to find enough qualified workers for the growing number of "knowledge jobs." A number of employers are addressing the deficiencies that many employees have in basic literacy and mathematical skills by administering basic skills assessments to employees. Then they conduct basic mathematics and English skills training classes at workplace sites for employees with deficiencies. Some employers also sponsor programs for employees and their family members to aid them in obtaining general equivalency diplomas. To address the skills deficiencies, HR management must do the following:

- Assess more accurately the knowledge and skills of existing employees, as well as the knowledge and skills needed for specific jobs.
- Make training for future jobs and skills available for employees at all levels, not just managers and professionals.
- Increase the usage of new training methods, such as interactive videos, individualized computer training, and via the Internet.
- Become active partners with public school systems to aid in upgrading the knowledge and skills of high school graduates.

GROWTH IN CONTINGENT WORKFORCE

In the past, temporary workers were used for vacation relief, maternity leave, or workload peaks. Today "contingent workers" (temporary workers, independent contractors, leased employees, and part-timers) represent over 20% of the workforce. Many employers operate with a core group of regular employees with critical skills and then expand and contract the Workforce through the use of contingent workers. This practice requires determining staffing needs and deciding in advance which employees or positions should form the "core" and which should be more fluid.

HUMAN RESOURCE MANAGEMENT POLICY

Human Resource Management, management strategy emphasizing the individual employee as against collective relations between management and labour. Human resource management (HRM) involves management relying less on hierarchy, instruction, and command; and, instead, becoming more participative and open. The aim is to promote cooperative relations between management and employees and to avoid the often adversarial behaviour associated with traditional industrial relations. Where HRM is successful, the employees will be committed to the long-term future of their organization and this, in turn, will help the organization adapt to competitive pressures.

HRM requires a package of measures including: employee involvement; relating pay to performance; care with selection and training and fair treatment of employees; and the dovetailing of personnel matters with other company policies such as production, marketing, and sales. Many organizations have one or a few of these elements but very few operate the whole package—so fully fledged HRM remains an unusual management style. HRM is not confined to any one sector.

There are three basic styles of employee-management relations. Traditionally, collective bargaining, where pay and conditions of employment are negotiated jointly between management and unions, has been the norm, but the coverage of such collectivism has been crumbling across the world. Secondly, in place of collective bargaining some organizations operate strong or weak forms of HRM. However, even more workplaces are authoritarian—the third basic style—characterized by managerial prerogative, with no trade union and no HRM.

Employee involvement requires providing employees with much more information than previously and consulting them more about the operation of the workplace. The key is two-way communication. Mere team briefings or cascading information down the management chain are not enough. Proper employee involvement means problem-solving groups such as quality circles, and regular meetings between top management and employees. Such communications emphasize the importance of quality control for the goods and services provided by the organization. Employee involvement permits the company to draw fully on the untapped knowledge, skills, and initiative of its employees. In this way, a high-trust relationship is fostered between management and labour.

Making pay contingent on performance is the second element of HRM. Instead of a common rate for the job, as happens with collective bargaining, pay varies according to the performance of the individual and of the firm. Employees are appraised and awarded individual performance-related pay. Profit-sharing and employee share schemes ensure that pay is also linked to the fortunes of the company. Under profit sharing a pay bonus is awarded according to the financial performance of the company. Employee share schemes provide some compensation in the form of shares that must be held for some years in the future. These help bind the employee to the company. Both profit sharing and employee share schemes mean that the company's workers are sharing both some of the risks and the benefits of the operation of the company with its owners.

Organizations operating HRM policies devote resources to staff recruitment, selection, appraisal, training, and development. They are particularly keen to employ individuals who can operate flexibly and adapt to different tasks as opposed to keeping to rigidly defined job demarcations. They must also be able to adapt to rapidly changing work arrangements such as annualized hours. These organizations would expect to eliminate old-fashioned hierarchies between white collar and blue collar workers. Employees would be treated similarly regarding method of payment, recording starting and finishing times, and subsidized meals.

The final element in HRM is that employee relations become the responsibility of all managers, not just personnel managers. More thought is also given to integrating personnel matters with the business functions of the company.

Three questions arise in evaluating HRM. Has it been implemented? Can unions survive in HRM organizations? What impact has HRM had on company performance? The various elements of HRM—employee involvement, contingent pay, emphasis on staff selection and development—are pervasive but they are usually introduced piecemeal rather than as a package. Indeed, unionized workplaces are more likely to have two-way communication methods and profit-sharing schemes than non-union workplaces. Any role for unions would be where the full package exists, radically different from that under traditional collective bargaining. For example, management would communicate directly with employees rather than via the union; pay would not be determined collectively but individually. This suggests a difficult time for unions in fully fledged HRM companies.

Where there is no union the collective representation of employees—as against consultation with individuals—becomes an important question. Some EU countries have works councils where labour and management meet, sometimes just for consultation, but in some countries to discuss, for example, investment strategy and the introduction of new technology. There is evidence that these works councils have a neutral or benign effect on company performance.

Evidence suggests that HRM workplaces have superior economic performance than authoritarian workplaces or those with collective bargaining. In particular, production levels and productivity growth are higher in HRM workplaces. By contrast, HRM does not generate good industrial relations. Resignations are higher, absenteeism is higher, and the climate of management-employee relations is worse in HRM workplaces than in other workplaces. This suggests that the "caring halo" sometimes associated with HRM is misplaced. This management system is designed to squeeze effort out of employees and commit them to the future performance of the company. Those that cannot stand the pace go absent or quit; and relations between managers and workers are tenser than is sometimes realized. But the system does deliver on the bottom line—it generates better economic outcomes.

THE CONCEPT OF HUMAN RESOURCE SYSTEM

HRM is a strategic approach to the acquisition, motivation, development and management of the organisation's human resources. It is a specialised field that attempts to divide an appropriate corporate culture, and introducing programmes which reflect and support the core values of the enterprise and ensure its success. HRM is proactive rather than reactive, i.e., always looking forward to what needs to be done and then doing it, rather than waiting to be told what to do about recruiting, paying or training people, or dealing with employee relations problems as they arise. The techniques for the application of HRM will include many familiar functions of personnel managers, such as manpower planning, selection, performance appraisal, salary administration, training and management development. These will be overlaid by special programmes designed to improve communication systems, involvement, commitment, and productivity. Broadly, there are three meanings attached to the concept of HRM. In the first place, persons working in an organization are regarded as a valuable source, implying that there is a need to invest time and effort in their development. Secondly, they are human resources which means that they have their own special characteristics and, therefore, cannot be treated like material resources. The approach focuses on the need to humanise organisational life and introduce human values in the organisation. And thirdly, human resources do not merely focus on employees as individuals, but also on other social realities, units and processes in the organisation.

These include the role or the job a person has in the organisation, the dyadic unit, (consisting of the person and his superior), the various teams in which people work, inter-team processes, and the entity of the total organisation. In its essence, HRM is the qualitative improvement of human beings who are considered the most valuable assets of an organization-the sources, resources, and end-users of all products and services. HRM is, no doubt, an outgrowth of the older process and approach. But it is much more than its parent disciplines viz., personnel management, and behavioural science. HRM is also more comprehensive and deep rooted than training and development. Its approach is multi-disciplinary from the beginning to the end.

It is a scientific process of continuously enabling the employees to improve their competency and capability to play their present as well as future expected roles so that the goals of the organization are achieved more fully and at the same time the needs of the employees are also met to an adequate extent. HRM is a production model approach to personnel management. The HRM model is characterised as being employee-oriented with an emphasis on the maximisation of individual skills and motivation through consultation with the workforce so as to produce high levels of commitment to company strategic goals. It is a resource to be used to its fullest capacity. It is an asset to be invested in.

HRM is concerned with both the structure of work in a firm and with all the related employment practices that are needed to carry out the work. HRM is not simply about HR or 'people practices', it is about the management of work and people in the firm. Managing people includes both individual and collective dimensions. The traditional personnel management is Non-strategic, separate from the business, reactive, short-term, and constrained by a limited definition of its role as dealing with mostly unionised and low level employees. The major attention of traditional personnel function is on personnel administration or management while the major attention of HRM is on developing people and their competencies. If personnel management is curative, HRM is preventive. The key distinguishing feature of HRM is its evolving strategic role. HRM essentially emphasises and incorporates those expectations which are not being fulfilled through the traditional personnel management.

It integrates in a meaningful way the various sub-systems like performance appraisal, potentiality appraisal and development, career planning, training and development, organisation development, research and systems development, rewards, employee welfare and quality of work life, industrial relations, and human resource information. Under the HRM approach, some basic assumptions about human resources are also different from the traditional approach. The important assumptions of HRM are as follows:

1) The members of an organisation are reservoirs of untapped resources.
2) There is scope for unlimited development of these resources.
3) It is more in the nature of self-development than development thrust from outside.
4) The organisation also undergoes development with the overall benefits along with the development of its members.
5) The organisation further develops a culture in which utmost emphasis is placed on harmonious superior-subordinate relations, teamwork, and collaboration among different groups of individuals, open communication, and above all, integration of the goals of the organisation with the needs of the employees.
6) Top management takes the initiative for HRM, formulates necessary plans and strategies, and creates an overall climate and support for its implementation.

The management of human resources is more of an art than a science. In practice it is an "art" full of pitfalls, judgment calls, and learning from past mistakes. Most employers and company owners agree the human resource department is one of the key components to the successfully running of their business. There are several aspects to the term "human resources". Here, we will discuss the human resource system, and why it is very important.

The human resource system can be defined as a core enterprise application which manages administrative and strategic processes related to the employees of a company. This complex, but imperative activity, is very important indeed for all human resources personnel.

The functions of the HR are many. It includes tracking and storing relevant information about the employee. Since this is a very long and tedious process, there was a need to reduce the workload on the human resource managers. Due to this, organizations automated many of the processes involved by introducing the human resource system.

The human resource system basically attempts to shape intersections between human resource management and information technology. It merges the HR management as a discipline, specifically with its basic processes and activities with the information technology arena.

The client server HR management systems are usually developed around four key components of HR functionalities. This includes payroll, administration, time, labour and human resources management. Products of the HR management system have been specifically designed to comprise of a series of modules which may be integrated to act as a single system, covering a wide range of functions, a part of human resources.

The HR management systems have proved to be a great success by significantly reducing the administrative burden on the human resources department. It also provides more convenient access to HR information, higher reporting functionality, more accurate and consistent data, superior internal profile, and standardized and efficient processes.

The HR systems allow for increasingly advanced functionality giving the companies an opportunity to get their routine transactions automated for line mangers, employees, and, of course, themselves.

The HR management systems are also credited for laying the foundation of e-HR strategy. This includes both e-learning and e-recruiting processes.

Choosing and implementing new HR systems is in itself a major project in terms of both time and money. It is the HR management's responsibility to ensure the system matches the core requirements of the department. The functionality of the system should be based on the naturalistic requirements of a particular organization.

But, because of the high capital involved in installing this application system, the HR systems are usually used only by medium and large companies. In such companies, the HR managers work with the internal software professionals to both develop and maintain the HR management systems.

The human resource system, however, are continuously evolving, and have now gone beyond their traditional functions to encompass many more HR fields and subjects, and therefore, needs to be upgraded accordingly

SYSTEM DESIGN IN HRD

Contextual Factors and System Designing

The main objectives of the design are:

1. Practicality
2. Efficiency
3. Cost
4. Flexibility
5. Security

System design contains Logical Design & Physical Designing, logical designing describes the structure & characteristics or features, like output, input, files, database & procedures. The physical design, which follows the logical design, actual software & a working system. There will be constraints like Hardware, Software, Cost, Time & Interfaces.

The processing techniques are

- Batch Processing
- Real-time
- Online
- Combination of all

Structured design is a data flow methodology. The graphical representation of data flow, communication & defining the modules & their relationship with each is known as Structure Chart. This method decomposes & modularizes the system so that the complexity & manageability will come down. Thus reducing the intuitive reasoning & promotes the maintainable provable systems.

This type of design follows top-down & hierarchy, which will have one single entry & single exit.

The advantages of this method are:

1. Critical interfaces are tested first
2. Early versions of the design, through incomplete are useful enough to resemble the real system
3. Structuring provides control & improve morale
4. The procedural characteristics define the order that determines processing.

Major System Design Activities are :-

1. DB design
2. Program design
3. System & program test prēparation
4. System Interface Specification
5. Audit Consideration
6. Audit control & Documentation control

Major design process parts are

1. O/p design
2. I/p design
3. File Design
4. Procedure design
   - Computer design
   - Non-computer design
5. Control design

These parts are inter-dependent on each other. **System Specifications** is a document, which will have a result of system design process, it serves as a Blue print for the project development & maintenance.

Prototype is a working system that is developed to test ideas & assumptions about a new system.

SUMMARY

Human Resource Development includes such opportunities as employee training, employee career development, performance management and development, coaching, succession planning, key employee identification, tuition assistance, and organization development. Human Resource Development can be formal such as in classroom training, a college course, or an organizational planned change effort. Or, Human Resource Development can be informal as in employee coaching by a manager. Healthy organizations believe in Human Resource Development and cover all of these bases. The elements of Human resource management planning are Planning and Appraisal, Individual and Team Development, Career Planning, Hiring, Career Pathing, Succession Planning, Job Design, Classification, Compensation /Recognition/Other Rewards. Goals and action plans of HRMP are Planning and Appraisal, Individual and Team Development, Career Planning Hiring, Career Pathing, Succession Planning, Job Design, Classification, Compensation/ Recognition/Other Rewards. HRM is not simply about HR or 'people practices', it is about the management of work and people in the firm. Managing people includes both individual and collective dimensions.

System design contains Logical Design & Physical Designing; logical designing describes the structure & characteristics or features, like output, input, files, database & procedures. Training and development encompasses three main activities: training, education, and development. Commonwealth organizations such have been at the forefront of work internationally in areas like teacher training, agricultural and health education, and in technical and vocational training.

UNIT 2

HUMAN RESOURCE PLANNING

INTRODUCTION

HR Planning for a business enterprise needs a conceptual outlay to enable business managers to identify, plan and implement planning for manpower. There is a need to appreciate basic definitions of planning as is understood and applied in commercial situations, the core strategy necessary for an organization to embark upon the journey of recruiting, the methods and practices adopted by organizations in a current scenario and the inherent constraints built into the planning process.

HR planning may be defined as an articulated business strategy based on current and future business forecast for the acquisition, utilization, development, and retention of an enterprise's human resources. The strategy articulates the need as it exists today and the plan necessitates formulation of the goals and action plan for achievement of the people plan. The process facilitates hiring and retaining the right profile of people at varying jobs, positions, places and time frames depending on the organizational need.

While considerable strategic time, competence and managerial inputs has been dedicated to the planning of corporate economic resources, such as investment, technology, systems, manufacturing capabilities, research and development, new product development, customer management, planning for resource requirement has been denied its priority, particularly at the company level. At the global level, manpower research are periodically organized more to determine employment potential, state of the unemployment rate, type, kind, demographics, rather than to identify, indicate and suggest on how the manpower requirements of the various priority areas and nations at large should be met, both qualitatively and quantitatively.

HR planning being a relatively contemporary activity, is today an area of in depth study and research. Its importance and implications, given the critical need for funding micro and macro level growth a fast changing economy, have been realized at the corporate level in most countries of the world. At the macro level, however despite the realization of the advantages of HR planning, countries with well-established HR planning programs are still a relative minority, even among the large countries. The ability to predict, plan, search, resource and execute a well orchestrated HR Plan is still not a state of art activity. Needless to mention the growing population in several parts of the world make this job several times more complex.

However on balance there is little evidence to claim that with the rising state of unemployment, several economies stagnating or into recession, increasing cost of labor and the substantial portion that it forms of the total running costs of a company, many more firms- large, medium and small- will be persuaded to go in for some of scientific HR planning. Fundamentally the market has changed. It is world of the knowledge worker. The rise of the intellect has been imminent. HR Planning no longer can confine itself to the traditional sources for hiring and retaining. The skill of yesterday is neither available and nor are not being sought after by the new generation. The human resources of today see their roles having changed from that of a doer to that of a thinker and in most occasions' thinker doer. Organizations in contrast have continued to nurture and retain a set of human resource who have become more redundant than ever before.

HR PLANNING: PURPOSE AND GOALS

The purpose and goals of HR planning are mainly:

1. *To ensure optimum and effective use of human resources currently employed*
2. *To research and reconfigure new skill sets to cope with organizational needs given depleting relevant skills population*
3. *To assess the employability of the human resource given changing skills and competencies*

4. *To draw specific outlines of competencies as they differ from today*
5. *To assess or forecast future skills requirement if organization's overall objectives are to be achieved and*
6. *To identify control standards to ensure that necessary resources are identified, available as and when required.*
7. *To fundamentally study the corporate strategy, the business mission and overall philosophy of recruiting VS systems, technology, outsourcing.*
8. *Analyze the people market environment and its changes as it affects the firm Vis a Vis competition.*

Corporate goals for attaching importance to HR planning and forecasting exercises are:

1. to determine hiring pattern and specific action plans
2. to anticipate redundancies
3. to minimize downsizing, surpluses, early retirement;
4. to plan for optimum training levels;
5. to manage management development programs;
6. new project forecasting and recruitment planning
7. to cost the manpower in new project;
8. to assist productivity bargaining; and
9. to assess future accommodation requirements.

PLANNING AHEAD FOR RECRUITMENT THE BASIC PROCESS OF HR PLANNING

1. Analyze the environment of the organisation and its past operations
2. Evaluate the environment for HR trends, patterns, educational changes, literacy levels, demographic transitions in people
3. Evaluate education patterns, school pass out rates, professional courses capacity, market liberalization for international opportunities, availability of easy financing for college studies
4. Evaluate any major shift in people relocation, geographic movements, natural calamity constraints

5. Establish Corporate strategy, goals, objectives and action plans
6. Link the corporate strategy to the HR strategy and mission
7. Ensure connectivity of corporate plans to hr plans and targets
8. Determine the Organisation Structure, process flows, design details
9. Draw up a Demand Forecast for Manpower
10. Conduct a HR Inventory both at the micro and macro levels
11. Plan for an Attrition Process both desired and undesired
12. Design HR policies for retention and career planning of high performers
13. Integrate HR policies with changing aspirations of the employees and the potential population in the market place
14. Draw up a supply Forecast for Manpower evaluating source, actual availability, possibility of attraction to the corporate
15. Study whether Demand is greater or less than Supply
16. Establish Manpower Objectives for short, medium and long term and keep a flexibility on the profile and employee fit with the corporate culture
17. Start an Action program and make individuals and teams responsible for meeting the recruitment targets.
18. Update the Manpower records and make system data friendly

STRATEGIC ADVANTAGES FOR HR PLANNING

There are a number of more specific reasons for resorting to HR planning exercises at the level of the undertaking, reasons that can make the exercise essential. These are:

1. *To establish the best cost balance between plant and manpower utilization.*
2. *To determine recruitment, level wise and occupation wise*
3. *Ensure that we do not inherit surplus manpower hired on account of an incompetent CEO.*
4. *To ensure that people do not substitute systems and process*
5. *To anticipate redundancies and avoid unnecessary dismissals or aspirations*

6. *To decide optimum training levels.*
7. *To decide on worker training courses*
8. *To provide a basis for management development programs*

MICRO/MACRO LEVEL ADVANTAGES

At the micro-level, corporate need to realize that manpower is a expensive and a highly valuable resource to be used as effectively as possible. Scientific level HR planning at the corporate level will make national planning more realistic and effective. The need for HR planning at all levels needs no mean emphasis.

Manpower planning at the national level will ensure that the human resources are made available both in quality and quantity for the planned development of the economic growth of the country. In our country, there has been considerable progress in this direction.

KEY POINTS FOR SUCCESSFUL HR PLANNING

HR planning must be recognized as an integral part of overall business planning. Hr planning should be lead by the CEO as his core responsibility. The manpower planner needs to know the company's objectives in terms of sales, marketing and growth. Top management backing and involvement for manpower planning is essential and should receive its rightful place hierarchically. The HR planning responsibility should be developed in consultation with line managers and their representatives. The forecast period should be prepared by skill levels rather than by aggregates of workers. Both the forecasting techniques, and the forecasts themselves, need to be constantly revised and improved in the light of experience.

CONCLUSION

Human resource is a key economic resource, and a scare one. It therefore demands the same attention a company gives to planning sales, investment or profits. It is this fact that has led to the development of manpower planning among an increasing number of business organizations. For the company, the returns from manpower planning can be measured in term of higher efficiency and productivity as a result of better utilization of its manpower resources and the elimination of waste in recruitment, training and other personnel schemes. The benefits to the individual employee and the country are not less important.

It is clear that a company cannot hope to forecast accurately its future manpower requirements unless these are related to future production and sales levels. The best results, therefore are achieved when a company has integrated HR planning with overall planning team is basically two fold: to interpret the forecasts for production and sales interns and manpower constraints on account of company policy for the future.

Four points need to be emphasized above the forecasting methods discussed in this note.

1. No Corporate can realistically accept evidence resulting from mechanical forecasting methods without a superimposing view on the macroeconomic environment.
2. The possibility of judgement done by individuals or groups performing the research is high and there is always room for the subjective/objective or intuitive assessment that the experienced manager can provide, only if needed.
3. In HR forecasting as in any other form of forecasting it is essential to recognize the wide margin of possible error, and therefore, preferable to think more in terms of a range of possible levels of demand for manpower, than of a single 'correct' estimate. The estimates need to be correlated to assumptions that are valid and proven. Futuristic assumptions need careful thought and research/ analysis.
4. Though the different analytical methods are presented as though they were alternatives, in practice a single company may wish to use two or more of them in different circumstances, as a check on one another. Finally it is abundantly evident that everything depends on the accuracy of the sales and output forecasts and the soundness of the calculations of turnover and wastage. The first task of a company must, therefore, be to ensure that the estimates are as reliable as possible.

Finally HR planning is continuous, ongoing process; and companies that treat it as a five-year burdensome task will be deeply disappointed. In fact it is preferable that they do start this task as it may turn into a ritual. Even the most carefully calculated forecasts are liable to be overtaken by unforeseeable changes. A system of assorting plans to these changes with as little delay as possible is an essential part of manpower planning. Indeed one might say that it is the essential characteristic of a well-managed enterprise. HR planning is a recruitment start up. HR planning is not the job of Human Resources Management (Personnel) people. It is the job of the CEO. Wherever the CEO has relinquished his responsibility and delegated HR hiring and structuring the organizations have lived to tell a tale. Corporate who seek the best minds to remain competitive need to plan for their hiring and thereafter their retention need to get their act together now. Absence of HR planning would mean an absence of a leader at a point in time now known now, definitely in the near future.

What is Functional Planning?

A functional plan essentially manages the work of a department that is concerned with performing the same type of work for all projects as well as performing non-project work. For project related work, the functional plan:

– ***Defines tasks at the level they can be assigned to an individual.***

Individuals in a functional organization must have a clear and unambiguous understanding of their work assignments.

– ***Produces clearly defined final outputs to other functional organizations.***

Clearly defined outputs helps ensure that needs of the program are satisfied, and the functional organization has a consistent checkpoint for measuring throughput of deliverables across the entire portfolio of programs.

– ***Tracks internal deliverables.***

Outputs that are never delivered to another functional activity or reported at the program level may nevertheless be important in order to move work *within* an organization.

– ***Includes a process for incorporating program requirements.***

A functional plan must "understand" when deliverables are required by a program, which deliverables are shared by multiple programs, and which program requirements are most restrictive at any particular time.

– ***Includes a process for managing competing priorities from multiple programs.***

Functional resources may often be strained to capacity when many programs compete for attention. Functional planning must incorporate processes that ensure the right program gets the right work done at the right time, and each program must also understand its position in the priority.

– ***May be impacted by non-project related work.***

Functional planning may be impacted by internal departmental activity such as training, process improvement initiatives, or other internal "projects".

– ***Includes change work***

Functional plans must also devote resources to managing changes to existing work products. For example, product designs are often revised as a result of new cost initiatives, test results or redesign of nearby components.

– ***Includes a process for assessing plan status***

Functional planners must have clearly defined processes for statusing work as complete. This is particularly important in the case of external deliverables.

In short, functional planning supports the work, costs, and resources of a particular department. This plan is often managed within the context of an overall program plan, but must also consider competing priorities from multiple programs, as well as internal initiatives and priorities such as process improvements and training requirements.

What is Cross-functional Planning?

Cross-functional planning brings together the activities of various functional groups in support of a single project. In the automotive industry, these projects are product development programs, whether the product is an entire vehicle or a sub-system or component.

Whereas functional planning focuses on moving work through the organization, cross-functional planning focuses on moving work from functional organization to functional organization. Given this objective, cross-functional planning will focus on managing the external outputs of a function -the key hand-offs between functions. Cross-functional planning can be summarized as follows:

– ***Work carried out by a single functional organization can be represented as a single activity***

The internal deliverables of a functional plan or schedule are not appropriate within the cross-functional plan. They are not the primary focus of the plan, which is to move work between departments. In cases where multiple deliverables are produced, additional activities may be included. For example, three major iterations of a product design may each be tracked, even though the work is performed by a single organization.

– ***Completion of an activity represents a hand-off to another organization***

This hand-off is required for the downstream functional group to either begin work, continue work or complete work. For example, the product design is required to begin developing the part tools.

– ***Includes a process for establishing program requirements***

The requirements passed down to a functional plan must meet the needs of the program, but it must also represent any initial trade-offs made among different functional groups. This allows the functional groups to share the risk inherent in any program plan by distributing any available float time equitably among the deliverable-producing functional group and the deliverable-using functional group.

– ***Focuses on planned activity***

Whereas the functional plan considers change work, the cross-functional focuses on Planned work. Taking the example of a product design, the cross-functional plan would track the initial product design only and ignore the ongoing revisions. The timing impact of those revisions will of course manifest themselves in longer tooling times.

– ***Includes a process for assessing the impact of plan status***

Understanding the status of activity progress is key to both functional and cross functional planning. For cross-functional plan, however, the focus is on understanding the impact to downstream activities in order, for example, to develop recovery plans. Where practical, cross-function plans should interface to functional schedules to obtain activity status.

EDUCATION AND DEVELOPMENT PLANNING

An Education Development Plan (EDP) documents an ongoing process in which a learner identifies both career goals and a plan of action to achieve them. The purpose of the EDP is to provide every student with a periodically updated and ongoing record of career planning that will guide in taking effective steps to enter a career of choice. Each student develops a first EDP in middle school, stating an initial career goal and desired work and educational experiences. School counsellors verify that EDPs reflect an individual career decision-making process based on career exploration, career assessment information, school performance, and expressed interests. School counsellors also facilitate selection and enrolment into general courses and into specialized education and training related to the career pathway of choice indicated in the EDP. Community colleges provide the opportunity to continue this planning process through EDP development.

Education Development Plan Standard and Benchmarks Standard

The participating education agency board of education or designee will have adopted for use in the district an Education Development Plan (EDP) to document student educational and career plans that encompasses the following six basic EDP elements approved by the Michigan Department of Career Development as part of the Career Preparation System: 1) personal information, 2) career pathway goals, 3) educational/training goals, 4) career assessment results, 5) plan of action, and 6) parent/family consultation and endorsement (under age 18).

Benchmarks

- The local board of education or designee has adopted Education Development Plans (EDP) that meet the state standard.
- Ensures that all middle school and high school buildings within the district utilize the Education Development Plan document and process adopted by the district as evidenced by student records in each building.
- Ensures that all students are engaged in developing initial EDPs before leaving the 8th grade level as evidenced by student records.
- Ensures that all high school students review and have opportunities to revise or update their EDPs at least annually to reflect changes in career decisions for use in selecting courses and in choosing post-secondary options as evidenced by guidance/ counselling plans and student records.

System design contains Logical Design & Physical Designing, logical designing describes the structure & characteristics or features, like output, input, files, database & procedures.

HUMAN RESOURCE DEVELOPMENT MECHANISMS

In order to fully appreciate the mechanisms for planning and implementation of HRD policies and programmes it is necessary to understand the planning budgeting and implementation mechanisms currently in operation in India. India being a Union of States, the responsibility for provision of the various components of HRD such as Education, Health, etc., are shared between the Central and State Governments. The State Governments who are the primary implementing agencies in most of the areas comprising HRD determine their own policies and also draw up their five year and annual plan of development. The Central Government, however, has a coordination and leading role in guiding the State policies and also in initiating national level programmes in crucial areas and in developing and ensuring national standards. The Central Government also provides substantial financial assistance to the States.

The Plans submitted by the State Governments under different sectors are coordinated by the Planning Commission headed by the

Prime Minister assisted by full time members and a team of professional staff. The Planning Commission has the responsibility for the scrutiny of the five year and annual plans of the States and the Centre ensuring finalisation of the Plans within the available resources and keeping in view national priorities. The Planning Commission works in close cooperation with the concerned Ministerial and the State Governments.

The Planning Commission currently has a full time Member-Charge of Human Resource Development. He looks after Education, Culture, Women & Child Development, Youth Services & Sports, besides Health and Social Welfare.

Hence at the level of Planning Commission there is a mechanism for coordination of many of the components of H.R.D. particularly the relating to the social sector and quality of life. Also the Member in charge of H.R.D. works in close cooperation with other members who are in charge of Science & Technology, Employment, Agriculture, Rural Development, etc., In a sense, therefore, the Planning Commission thus becomes an effective coordinating agency for H.R.D. As it is charged with the responsibility of developing perspective long term plans as wall as mid-term plans and annual plans and is also responsible for evaluation and mentoring, the planning Commission is in a unique position to ensure the development of H.R.D. and to monitor their implementation.

Its coordination, however, is confined to policy and planning aspects, The executive responsibility for formulating H.R.D. policies and their implementation vests with a number of administrative Ministries. The most important among them from of point of view is the Ministry of H.R.D. This Ministry comprises the Departments of Education, Culture, Youth Services & Sports, and Women & Child Development. A Cabinet level Minister is in charge of the entire Ministry. He is assisted by two State Ministers; one in charge of Education & Culture and another in charge of Youth Services & Sports, and Women & Child Development. The Minister is assisted by a full time Secretary for Human Resource Development whose task is, inter alia, to coordinate the work of four independent Departments each with a full time Secretary, Similarly in some of the States similar mechanism has been set up with a full time Secretary for H.R.D.

Co-ordinating the work of Education, Health etc. However, it may be noted that there is no effective mechanism as yet developed for coordination between Education, and Employment Science and Technology, Rural Development etc. One of the important tasks ahead is the development of H.R.D. programme after due coordination with all the Departments concerned with this task.

Within the Ministry of H.R.D. a certain measure of coordination has been attempted. As pointed out by Mid-term Appraisal of the 7th Five Year Plan a major theme of the 7th Plan is the integration of H.R.D. programmes with other programmes. Some progress has been made towards this. Firs integration between different activities within the sector has been promoted e.g. between health care and family welfare; Second, integration between health, education and related sectors has been pursued e.g. between child-care and pre-primary education, between education health and nutrition in the integrated Child Health Care and enrolment and retent— in the school health programme. Third, human resource development is being integrated with other development activities e.g. by use of National Rural Employment Programme etc.

The executive responsibility for human resource development at a national level is now shared by the Ministry of H.R.D. with other Ministries such as Ministry of Labour which is responsible for technical training of workers, the Department of Health which is responsible for the provision of health services, the Department of Science & Technology and indeed several other In statutes working in this area. Mention must be made of the Institute of Applied Manpower

Research with its programmes in the area of man-power and human resource development. A Cabinet Committee an H.R.D. has also been set up recently. Thus while it is true that there is no tingle agency which is responsible for all H.R.D. programmes a strong lead has been taken in this regard by the Ministry of H.R.D., which has sought to establish linkages with all other departments and agencies concerned with H.R.D.

As already stated similar arrangements exist at the State level in a number of States wherein Secretaries have be designated as in charge of H.R.D. But it is not adequate to have nodal agencies coordinating H.R.D. programmes at Central and State levels only. The major requirement is that of coordination at the cutting edge of implementation namely, in the villages and blacks. The Seventh Plan has pointed out that over the years the delivery system particularly in regard to social services has not been able to obtain effectiveness as originally envisaged. The position varies among the State but an almost uniform feature has been the gradual erosion of the control of the Block Development Officer over the extension team at the block and village levels. Simultaneously, a multiplicity of functionaries has emerged at this level for implementation of a large number of programmes aimed at the same people for raising their standard of living. Similarly, Panchayati Raj institutions in one form or another exist in most States but they have not been effectively involved in the implementation or rural development programmes. Where they are so involved quality programme implementation has be decidedly better.

With the launching of the large scale multi-sectoral country-wide programmes of rural development aiming both at individual households and at the creation of assets in the rural areas the original concept of community Development could be said to have been substantially restored. This would be further strengthened by the measures already taken to rationalise the administration and delivery mechanism.

What goes by the name of Community Development will have to be viewed more in the nature of a scheme for village development which would imply the planning and implementation of a number of residual activities the village level which does not get covered in the norm sectoral plans and special programmes. This in turn will have to be on the basis of local decentralised planning at the village and block levels for which both in the nature of outright and incentive grants, would have to be placed at the disposal of panchayati Raj and Community Development bodies rather than by forming sectoral plans for the villages at the state and National levels. This would imply a considerable degree of rationalisation in the drawing up plans for community Development and Panchayati Raj and substantial autonomy in their implementation.

In addition States would be called upon to active Panchayati Raj institutions particularly at the village and block levels with a view to ensure their active involvement in the planning and development.

HUMAN RESOURCE PROCESSES

Every method or mechanism has two dimensions: **substantive and procedural**. Substantive dimension is what is being done; process is how it is accomplished, including how people are relating to each other and what processes and dynamics are occurring. In most of the organisations there is overemphasis on the substantive aspect of method and the procedural aspect is neglected. Whenever there is a problem in the organisation its solution is sought in the rules and structures rather than in the underlying group dynamics and human behaviour. Thus, rules may be changed, structure may be modified but group dynamics and human behaviour remain unfortunately untouched. It is thought that there is no need to pay any attention to them. This is wrong. In every organisation human process must receive as much importance (if not more) as the substantive dimension. One can find six such processes in operation in an organisation at six different levels HRD methods help in improving these processes as described below:

1. At the personal level there is the existential process. This process tells us how an individual perceives his environment, how he interacts with others, how he achieves his goals in life and so on. If this process is neglected it may adversely affect the integration of the individual with organisation and his quality of work. Career Planning, Performance Appraisal and Review, Feedback, Counselling, Job Enrichment, objective rewards, etc., improve this process.
2. At the interpersonal level we have the empathic process. This process tells us how much empathy one individual has for the other person and how does he reach out to the other person and establishes a relationship with him. Communication, conflict, cooperation and competition are some important areas of study

in this process. If this process is neglected it may adversely affect the interpersonal effectiveness of individuals in an organisation. Training, Rotation, Communication, etc., improve this process.

3. At the role level we have the coping process. Every individual is required to cope with various pressures and stresses in relation to his role in the organisation. However, if the individual's role is clear and the individual is aware of the competencies required for role performance he can cope with these pressures effectively. Role analysis goes a long way to improve this process.
4. At the group level we have the building process. This process tells us how various groups form themselves as distinct entities in an organisation; how do they become cohesive while the substantive (or structural) dimension has its grounding in classic] organisation theory the procedure/dimension reflects the human relations movement and strong and how can they effectively contribute to the goals of the organisation. Several team-building exercises improve this process.
5. At the intergroup level we have the collaborative and the competitive processes. Both can be either positive or negative. Competition is positive if it poses a challenge to a group in terms of standard of performance and achievement. It is negative if it prevents a group from attaining its goals. Similarly, collaboration is positive if it aims at helping others in achieving a common goal. It is negative if it aims at escaping hard work. This process can be very much improved by creating a climate of trust, authenticity, openness etc. and by clarifying norms and standards.
6. At the organisational level we have the growth process, which involves issues relating to organisational climate, self-renewal and change. To enhance the efficiency of human resource management, Indian corporate are now increasingly resorting exploring an increasingly popular technique called "Process Mapping" (PM). According to experts, it's a technique of doing away with non-value adding activities in key people management processes such as recruitment, training and development and team management. Such 'non-priority' activities or processes

are hived off so that the companies can consolidate an efficient people management system that can enable HR in contributing better to business strategy.

And the reasons behind PM gaining currency as a strategic Human Resource Management (HRM) tool in corporate India are legion. Consultants inform that PM aids in cutting the cycle time in various initiatives in people management across domains, thereby optimising the time and cost of the organisation. As Mr. Jacob J, senior consultant, Feedback Ventures, an HR consultancy puts it: "The constant focus in Process Mapping is to shrink the time and speed-up a whole gamut of HR initiatives". Further, it also enables the organisation to rationalise manpower and create a leaner enterprise. This is because when the corporate hive off the insignificant processes the manpower attached to those processes also move out with that. Another reason for PM gaining prominence is that it also aids companies in creating certain benchmarked HR systems. This is because PM is also about analysing every individual step in an initiative and finding ways to refine them.

HUMAN RESOURCE DEVELOPMENT OUTCOMES

Following are the various outcomes, which result from HRD methods via improvement in the human processes:

1. People in the organisation become more competent because on the one hand they become better aware of the skills required for job performance and on the other hand there is greater clarity of norms and standards.
2. People understand their roles better because through increased communication they become aware of the expectations, which other members of their role set have from them.
3. People become more committed to their jobs because now there is greater objectivity in the administration of rewards. They come forward with better and more creative ideas.
4. People develop greater trust and respect for each other. They become more open and authentic in their behaviour. Thus new values come to be generated.

5. There is greater collaboration and teamwork, which produces synergy effect.
6. People find themselves better equipped with problem solving capabilities. They become more prone to risk-taking and proactive in their orientation. There is greater readiness on their part to accept change.
7. Lot of useful and objective data on employees are generated which facilitate better human resource planning.
8. The top management becomes more sensitive to employees' problems and human processes due to increased openness in communication. The net result of the above outcomes is that the organisation becomes more effective. It achieves new heights in terms of productivity, cost, growth, diversification, profits and public image. However, one should not expect these results in a short period. But if these results do not appear even after a reasonably long period one should question the qualitative and quantitative adequacy of the HRD processes and the related instruments which are being used in that organisation. It should also be remembered that excellent HRD outcomes at any given point of time do not indicate continued effectiveness of the organisation for all times to come. HRD results need to be continuously watched, strengthened and renewed. Over the years, researchers have collected a fair amount of empirical evidence that certain HRD practices can directly affect an organization's performance

HRD Program evaluation is the final phase in the training and HRD process. This is where the effectiveness of the HRD intervention is measured. This is an important but often ignored activity. Careful evaluation provides information on participants' reaction to the program, how much they learned, whether they use what they learned back on the job, and whether the program improved the organization's effectiveness. HRD professionals are increasingly being asked to provide evidence of the success of their efforts using a variety of "hard" and "soft" measures, that is, both bottom line impact, as well as employee reaction. This information allows, managers to make better decisions about various aspects of the HRD effort, such as:

- Continuing to use a particular technique or vendor in future programs
- Offering a particular program in the future
- Budgeting and resource allocation
- Using some other HR or managerial approach (like employee selection or Changing work rules) to solve the problem.

It is important that HRD professionals provide evidence that HRD programs improve individual and organizational effectiveness. Armed with this information, HRD managers can better compete with managers from other areas of the organization when discussing the effectiveness of their actions and competing for resources.

ACTIVITY ANALYSIS

Identification and description of activities in an organization, and evaluation of their impact on its operations. Activity analysis determines (1) what activities are executed, (2) how many people perform the activities, (3) how much time they spend on them, (4) how much and which resources are consumed, (5) what operational data best reflects the performance of activities, and (6) of what value the activities are to the organization. This analysis is *accomplished* through direct observation, *interviews*, *questionnaires*, and *review* of the *work records*. See also *job analysis*, *performance analysis* and *task analysis*.

Activity Analysis and Development is a framework for studying and developing work activities, particularly in relation to information systems development. It is based on *Developmental Work Research*, which in turn is an application of *Activity Theory* on work development.

TASK ANALYSIS

'Task analysis is the analysis of how a *task* is accomplished, including a detailed description of both manual and mental activities, task and element durations, task frequency, task allocation, task complexity, environmental conditions, necessary clothing and equipment, and any other unique factors involved in or required for one or more people to perform a given task. Task analysis emerged from research in *applied behavior analysis* and still has considerable research in that area.

Information from a task analysis can then be used for many purposes, such as *personnel selection* and *training*, tool or equipment design, *procedure* design (e.g., design of *checklists* or *decision support systems*) and *automation*.

The term "task" is often used interchangeably with *activity* or *process*. Task analysis often results in a hierarchical representation of what steps it takes to perform a task for which there is a goal and for which there is some lowest-level "action" that is performed. Task analysis is often performed by *human factors* professionals.

Task analysis may be of manual tasks, such as bricklaying, and be analyzed as *time and motion studies* using concepts from *industrial engineering*. Cognitive task analysis is applied to modern work environments such as *supervisory control* where little physical works occurs, but the tasks are more related to *situation assessment*, *decision making*, and response planning and execution.

Task analysis is also used in *education*. It is a model that is applied to classroom tasks to discover which *curriculum* components are well matched to the capabilities of students with *learning disabilities* and which task modification might be necessary. It discovers which tasks a person hasn't mastered, and the information processing demands of tasks that are easy or problematic. In behavior modification, it is a breakdown of a complex behavioral sequence into steps. This often serves as the basis for *Chaining*.

REWARD MANAGEMENT

Reward system usually means the financial reward on organization gives its employees in return for their labour. While the term, reward system, not only includes material rewards, but also non-material rewards. The components of a reward system consist of financial rewards (basic and performance pay) and employee benefits, which together comprise total remuneration. They also include non-financial rewards (recognition, promotion, praise, achievement responsibility and personal growth) and in many case a system of performance management. Pay arrangements are central to the cultural initiative as they are the most tangible expression of the working relationship between employer and employee. Many papers examine the role of organizational culture i.e., the demand for mentoring compensation. Such investigations conclude that organizational culture places a significant role in determining the level of economic demands. Recent researches on industrial unrest rest indicate that reward criteria of the organisations both financial and non-financial rewards have tremendous influence upon the employees and employers performance.

These components will be designed, developed and maintained on the basis of reward strategies and policies which will be created within the context of the organizations between strategies, culture and environment: they will be expected to fulfil the following broad aims;

1. **Improve Organizational Effectiveness**: Support the attainment of the organization's mission, strategies, and help to achieve sustainable, competitive advantage.
2. **Support and change culture**: Under pin and as necessary help to change the 'organizational culture' as expressed through its values for performance innovation, risks taking, quality, flexibility and team working.
3. **Achieve Integration**: Be an integrated part of the management process of the organization. This involves playing a key role in a mutually reinforcing and coherent range of personal policies and process.
4. **Supportive Managers**: Support individual managers in the achievement of their goals.
5. **Motivate Employees** : Motivate employees to achieve high levels of quality performance.
6. **Compete in the Labour Market**: Attract and retain high quality people.
7. **Increased Commitment**: Enhance the commitment of employees to the organization that will a) want to remain members

of it, b) develop a strong belief in and acceptance of the values and goals of the organization and c) be ready and willing to exert considerable effort on its behalf.

8. **Fairness and Equity**: Reward people fairly and consistently according to their contribution and values to the organization.
9. **Improved Skills**: Upgrade competence and encourage personal development.
10. **Improved Quality**: Help to achieve continuous improvement in levels of quality and customer service.
11. **Develop team working**: Improve co-operation and effective team working at all level.
12. **Value for money**: Pride value for the money for the organization.
13. **Manageable**: Be easily manageable so that undue administrative burdens are not imposed on managers and members of the personal department.
14. **Controllable**: Be easily controllable so that the policies can be implemented consistently and costs can be contained within the budget.

Intrinsic rewards

Intrinsic rewards are less tangible, originate from persons or job it and reflect Herzberg motivators. Example of such factors includes;

- Variety in Job Content.
- Sense of being a part of value adding process.
- Believe that they are valuable members of a team.
- Increased responsibility and autonomy.
- Sense of accomplishment.
- Participation in setting targets and opportunities to achieve them.
- Feedback information.
- Recognition.
- Opportunities to learn and grow.

Extrinsic rewards

Results from the actions of others, such as supervisions are more easily controlled by managers. Examples include pay, fringe benefits, praise and promotion.

Meaning of reward to people

Pay is frequently used as a motivator and reinforce on it can easily be differentiated and computed, linked, clearly and visibly to direct performance and is generally valued reward. While outlined the major components in the meaning of reward to people;

- Short-term material enjoyment.
- Long term security,
- Social status.
- Recognition of personal achievement.

SUMMARY

HR planning may be defined as an articulated business strategy based on current and future business forecast for the acquisition, utilization, development, and retention of an enterprise's human resources. Human resource is a key economic resource, and a scare one. It therefore demands the same attention a company gives to planning sales, investment or profits. HR planning is continuous, ongoing process; and companies that treat it as a five-year burdensome task will be deeply disappointed. In order to fully appreciate the mechanisms for planning and implementation of HRD policies and programmes it is necessary to understand the planning budgeting and implementation mechanisms currently in operation in India. Substantive dimension is what is being done; process is how it is accomplished, including how people are relating to each other and what processes and dynamics are occurring. Over the years, researchers have collected a fair amount of empirical evidence that certain HRD practices can directly affect an organization's performance. HRD Program evaluation is the final phase in the training and HRD process. This is where the effectiveness of the HRD intervention is measured. Activity analysis determines (1) what activities are executed, (2) how many people perform the activities, (3) how much time they spend on them, (4) how much and which resources are consumed, (5) what operational data best reflects the performance of activities, and (6) of what value the activities are to the organization. Information from a task analysis can then be used for many purposes, such as *personnel selection* and *training*, tool or equipment design, *procedure* design (e.g., design of *checklists* or *decision support systems*) and *automation*. Reward system usually means the financial reward on organization gives its employees in return for their labour.

UNIT 3

TRAINING IN HUMAN RESOURCE DEVELOPMENT

INTRODUCTION

Human Resource is the backbone of any organization. Properly trained and highly skilled human resource is perceived as the greatest asset of an organization. Skilled personnel contribute to efficiency, growth, increased productivity and market reputation of an organization. This has been realized by industrial, commercial, research establishments and even governments. Invariably, a separate Human Resources Development department exists in all these organizations to attend to the matters relating to recruitment, training and deployment.

Technological advancements in various fields world over are very rapid, and the every other day we see new products or machines or equipments with more and more advanced features, with which users have to be acquainted. In order to cope with the industry demand and technological advancements, we need to develop training strategy for our human capital to attain the required skill levels.

Training is referred to as a method to give the new entrant or an existing employee the skills, knowledge and attitude needed to perform the job. Training should meet two basic objectives.

1. Training should make the personnel skilled enough to do the job on hand efficiently leading to targeted productivity levels.
2. Training should be cost effective.

Training must be based on scientific approach and quality training material to meet objective number one. The training duration should be as short as possible and resources used efficiently for meeting objective required.

What is training?

Training – refers to a planned effort by a company to facilitate employees' learning of job-related competencies

- The *goal of training* is for employees to:

Master the knowledge, skill, and behaviors emphasized in training programs, and apply them to their day-to-day activities.

High-Leverage Training

- Linked to strategic goals and objectives
- Uses an instructional design process to ensure that training is effective
- Compares or benchmarks the company's training programs against training programs in other companies
- Creates working conditions that encourage *continuous learning*

Continuous Learning

- Continuous Learning – requires employees to understand the entire work system including the relationships among:
  - their jobs
  - their work units
  - the entire company
- *Employees* are expected to:
  - acquire new skills and knowledge
  - apply them on the job
  - share this information with other employees
- *Managers* take an active role:
  - in identifying training needs
  - helping to ensure that employees use training in their work

Important Concepts in Training

- Knowledge
- Skill
- Attitude

- Knowledge
    - Knowledge - information we place into
    - memory - declarative (factual), procedural and strategic *(Kraiger et al 1993)*
- Knowledge: (for learning)
    - Information we acquire and place into memory
    - How information is organized for use into what we already knows
    - Our understanding of how, when and why information is used and is useful.

Phases of Learning a Skill

- Strategic Knowledge
- For planning, mentoring, and revising the goal directed activity.
- Skill - capacities needed to perform a set of tasks that are developed as a result of training and experience *(Dunnette 1976).*
- *Application of the facts already learned*

Transferable Skills for Communications, Sales/marketing

- Speaking and Listening effectively
- Creatively expressing ideas
- Negotiating
- Persuading
- Reporting information
- Describing feelings

Transferable Skills for Administrative Tasks

- Plan and arrange
- Bring order out of confusion
- Attention to detail
- Use of technology to organize and present information
- Flexibility: see obstacles as a challenge rather than a setback
- Manage multiple tasks

Transferable Skills for Organizational Leadership

- Initiating new ideas
- Handling details
- Delegating responsibility
- Teaching
- Coaching/Counseling
- Promoting change
- Decision making
- Managing conflict

Transferable Skills for Work Survival

- Cooperation
- Punctual
- Time Management
- Attention to detail
- Goals and Objectives
- Accepting responsibility
- Organizing
- Making decisions

General transferable skills

- *communication*: the ability to present an communicate in written and oral form and to use language appropriately in complex argument
- *problem-solving*: the ability to identify and analyze practical issues arising in a situation and to offer a practical solution, making effective use of time and resources available
- *teamwork*: the ability to establish working relations with others, to interact effectively, and to promote productive cooperation

General transferable skills

- *autonomy and personal skills*: the ability to act independently, to deal with the unexpected, to reflect on one's own actions and to accept and provide constructive feedback
- *information technology:* the ability to use IT tools and develop that use by integrating it into their own work

- *numeracy:* the ability to make use of numerical and statistical information as part of an argument or in a report
- *Intellectual skills*: the ability to analyze, think critically, evaluate and synthesize information.

Attitudes

- Attitudes - beliefs and opinions that support or inhibit behaviour *(Oskamp 1991) Towards management, trade union, empowerment, training, Job satisfaction, job stress*

Why Study Attitudes?

- Strongly influence our social thought Help to organize and evaluate stimuli (e.g., categorizing stimuli as positive or negative)
- Often have a strong affect on behavior Help to predict people's behavior in wide range of contexts (e.g., voting, interpersonal relations)
- Often they are ambivalent Evaluate object both positively and negatively
- To determine why they are so resistant to change Features
- Attitude affects behavior
- Attitudes are invisible
- Attitudes are acquired
- Attitudes are pervasive

Four Basic Attitude Functions

- Utilitarian - what it will do for you
- Ego defensive function - helps protect customer self image
- Value expressive - reflects customers general values, life-style or attitude
- Knowledge - cater to customer need to know

Role of Training

- Building employee capabilities
- Employee Orientation
- Newcomer Socialization
- Enterprise Training

- Building Team Effectiveness
- Developing Leaders

Forces Influencing the Workplace and Training

- Globalization
- Need for leadership
- Increased value placed on knowledge
- Attracting and retaining talent
- Customer service and quality emphasis
- Changing demographics and diversity of the work force
- New technology
- High-performance models of work systems
- Economic changes

Challenges for HRD

- Changing workforce demographics
- Competing in global economy
- Eliminating the skills gap
- Need for lifelong learning
- Need for organizational learning

Competing in the Global Economy

- New technologies
- Need for more skilled and educated workers
- Cultural sensitivity required
- Team involvement
- Problem solving
- Better communications skills

Need for Lifelong Learning

- Organizations change
- Technologies change
- Products change
- Processes change

- People must change

Need for Organizational Learning

- Organizations must be able to learn, adapt, and change
- Principles:
    - Systems thinking
    - Personal mastery
    - Mental models
    - Shared visions
    - Team learning

ORGANISATIONAL TRAINING

Organization and change

Beliefs (Old)

- The environment is stable and competitive no undue pressure for innovation
- Jobs are well defined and slow to change
- Employment relationships are long-term
- The psychological contract exchanges long-term security and gradual advancement for employee loyalty and sacrifice
- Workforces are relatively homogeneous
- Relatively little need for inter-group cooperation across different functional specialties

Beliefs (New)

- Unstable Environment
- Fast Changing Job Designs and Descriptions
- Specialization
- Uncertainty to job
- Heterogeneous Work Shop
- Self Managed Teams
- Competency
- Joint ventures, alliances and partnerships

Traditional & Emerging Paradigms: Forces on Organizations

Change and HRD

- Centralization to decentralization
- Individual effort to Team effort
- Long term to short term
- Vertical structure to Flat structure
- Autocratic to co-leadership
- Task intensive to labour intensive
- Soft culture to synergetic culture
- Localization to globalization
- Mass sizing to smart sizing
- Power orientation to relationship orientation
- Certainty to uncertainty

Challenges of HRD

- Philosophical Change - Ultimate understanding of HRD
- The Value Change - Regarding people, Human Beings and Ourselves
- Content Change - Substance, Teaching and Training
- The Challenge of Policy - In construction and structuring of realities.
- Economic and Technological Changes
- Shift in jobs for manufacturing and agriculture to service industries and telecommunications.
- Pressures of global competition causing firms to adapt by lowering costs and increasing productivity.
- Growth of information technology (Internet)

HRD

- It is the process by which the employees of an organization are helped in a continuous planned way to—Acquire or sharpen capabilities required to perform various functions associated with their present or expected or future roles.

- Develop their general capabilities as individuals and discover and exploit their inner potentials for their own and or organizational development purposes.
- Develop an organizational culture in which supervisor subordinates relationships, team work, and collaboration among subunits are strong and contribute to professional well being, motivation and pride of employees.

HRD Definition

- A set of systematic and planned activities designed by an organization to provide its members with the necessary skills to meet current and future job demands.

HRD Meaning

- To develop capabilities of each employees as an individual
- The capabilities of each individual in relation to his or her future role.
- The capabilities of each individual in relation to his or her expected future roles
- The dyadic relationship between each employee and his or her supervisor
- The team spirit and functioning in every organizational unit (Department, group)
- The organizational over all health and self renewing capabilities of individual's dyads, teams and entire organizations.

HRD and Training

Training

- In nut shell
  - A systematic and planned change
  - Learning process
  - Evaluation

Learning

- A continuous process in the work life of employees
- Leave no doubt in the mind of employees
- Will show up prospects for development of employees

- aims at bringing out improved and better employees
- Requires planning and setting up of goals or objectives and map out particular course through which the employees have to pass through to reach their goals
- Review is one of the essential feature of development process

According to Richard Calhoun – the process of aiding employees to gain effectiveness in their present and future work.

According to Dale S Beach – the organized procedure by which people learn knowledge and skill for a definite purpose.

According to Michael, Armstrong the systematic development of the knowledge, skill and attitudes required by an individual to perform adequately a given task or job.

A learning process by which people acquire, skills, concepts, attitudes or knowledge to aid in the achievement of goals – Robert L Mathis, and John H Jackson.

Training

It is any attempt to improve current or future employee performance by increasing an employees ability to perform through learning, usually, by changing the employees attitude or increasing his or her skills and knowledge.

Need for training

- The need for training and development is determined by the employees performance, deficiency computed as follows;
- Training and development need = standard performance – Actual performance
  - Individual level
  - Operational level
  - Organizational level

Managerial Skill gap: Marketing

- Technical skill (Comfortable with MS office, SPSS, SAS etc.)
- Communication skill (Fluency in English, good written and oral)
- Sales promotion skills

- Presentation skills
- Negotiation skills
- Convincing Skill
- Influencing skill
- Market Planning skill
- Organizing skill
- Network deployment skill
- Selling skills
- Personal selling skills
- Leadership skill (Team)
- Customer Relationship skills (CRM)
- Coordination skill
- Research skill
- Reporting skills
- Adaptive skill
- Problem solving skills
- Decision-making skills
- Coaching and developing skills
- Product planning and development skills
- Project management skill
- Ability to perform under stress
- Knowledge of marketing and sales software operations

Managerial Skill gap in HR

- Observation skill
- Analytical skill
- Decision making skill
- Problem solving skill
- Negotiation skill
- Coordination skill
- Communication skill

- Leadership skill
- Team building skill
- Conflict management skill
- Training skill
- Interviewing skill
- Networking skill
- Planning and organizing skill
- Research Skill
- Appraisal skill
- Computation skill
- Technical skill
- Change management skill
- Performance orientation skills
- Work orientation skills
- Value orientation skills
- Mentoring skills
- Coaching skills
- Counseling skills
- Talent management skill
- Policy Development skill
- Facility Management skill
- Relationship management skill

Managerial Skill gap in Finance

- Computation skills
- Analytical skills
- Decision making skill
- Problem solving skill
- Fund raising skills
- Wealth maximization skill (equity)
- Profitability maximization skill
- Asset management skill

- Risk management skill
- Investment management skill
- Financial planning skill
- Financial execution and control skill
- Security analysis skill
- Broking skill
- Portfolio development skill
- Financial trading skill
- Cash flow management skill
- Venture capital management skill
- Working capital management skill
- Cost accounting skills
- Management accounting skills
- Statistical analysis skill
- Tax management skill
- Reconciliation skill
- Budgeting skill
- Reporting skill
- Problem solving skill
- Decision making skill
- Presentation skill

Importance of training

- Improve employees skill and knowledge
- Enables them to develop within the organization
- To increase he out put qualitatively and quantitatively
- It ensures efficient and economical use of both equipment and materials in the plant Wastages are minimized
- It helps engaging managerial attention more towards planning than spending their valuable time in correcting the mistakes of the deficient employees
- It reduces the rate of absenteeism and Provides a little scope complaints and grievances

- It develops abilities to meet the challenges posed by organizational, social, and technological changes.
- A good investment in HR for long term return.

Aims and objectives of training

- Develop capacities and capabilities of employees
- New knowledge and new skills
- Training helps existing employees to improve their level of performance
- Create self consciousness and greater awareness to recognize their responsibilities to contribute best
- Open more vistas for promotion to more responsible job
- To reduce the employee turn over and keep the man power employment cost at the lowest level
- Apprenticeship training program aiming at improving the skills of present employers and come to the aid of the company to tide over tight labor market position
- To bring about efficiency and effectiveness in the organization
- To bring about congenial industrial relations where ever the companies undergo automation and technological change

Training outcome

- Improved productivity
- Higher out puts
- Morale
- Increased sales
- Faster and better coordination
- Health and safety
- Prevalent obsolescence
- Personnel growth
- Reduce dissatisfaction, complaints and grievances, absenteeism, turnover
- Better and more economical use of machines, equipments, and materials

- Minimum Wastages
- Lower unit costs

Benefits of Effective Management Education

- Exposure to new and better ideas and practices of application
- Motivate managers to improve performance
- Helps managers actually develop/improve skills
- Cause reflection, introspection and self appraisal
- Helps to identify specific performance problems
- Increase managers confidence
- Reduces the managerial stress
- Encourage to think differently
- Encourage career development planning
- Model to subordinates

Negative consequences of poorly trained managers

- Great difficulty in achieving performance goals
- Loss of employee productivity
- Loss of team work/cooperation/communication
- Morale problems/increased stress
- Loss of focus on customer needs and profitability
- Increased cost/lost opportunities
- Quality problems/unresolved performance barriers
- Absenteeism and turnover problems
- Broken policies and procedures/ potential legal exposure
- Bad habits develop

Failure of training in organization

- Training not a priority to top leadership
- Over reliance on trial and error learning
- Unwilling to take time to train/educate
- Assumes managers are already competent
- No accountability for MDP

- Reluctant to spent money
- Unclear management skill set
- Lack of formal management training process
- Assume Management Training is the managers responsibility
- Lack of qualified trainers

Organizational constraints

- Need high level of simulation
- Task is critical to the job
- Mistakes are costly
- Trainees vary in amount of experience
- Trainees have large differences in ability levels
- Mix of employees and new hires trained on a new procedure
- Long lag between end of training and use of skill on the job
- Short lead time
- Bias against a type of training
- Few trainees available at any one time
- Small organization with limited fund

Budgeting for training

Depends on various factors

Who

- Designers knowledge & skill
- Knowledge of the training subject
- Size and complexity of the target training group
- Clients track records for sticking to plan
    - Depends on various factors

What

- The number of instruction modules
- The elements included in the training materials
- Clients or organizations expectation regarding packaging
- What is considered the final product

How

- Data collection
- The designers interaction with the client
- The clients level of involvement
- The programmes degree of interactivity

Training programmes cost

- Direct cost
- Indirect cost
- Overhead cost
- Participant Compensation
- Evaluation cost

Direct cost

- Programme development cost
- Cost of TNA
- Cost evaluation
- materials and design
- Computer based programming
- Piloting of the programme
- Directly attributed to the delivery of the training programme
- Travel, materials (that could be used in future)
- Facilities, beverages, equipment rental and trainer compensation

Indirect cost

- Non-development items
- Trainer compensation for preparation
- Materials purchased/duplication (if not suitable in purchase)
- Marketing expenses
- Administrative and clerical support (Compensation rate for time spent on project) and
- Any materials already sent to trainees

Overhead cost

- General operating cost of the training programme

- Large organizations: programmes share of purchases and maintenances of training equipment, clerical, administrative support, training facilities etc.
- Small organizations: no over head costs are likely to be involved.

Participant Compensation

- Their salaries and benefits to be included as a cost of training
- Another way to approach this expense calculation is to include only the cost of replacing those employees, while they are in training
- When managers are taking out for training programme routine matter to be attended by some other managers

Evaluation cost

- Cost associated with evaluation of training
- Development of assessment tools
- Time spent administering tools
- Analyzing & preparing reports
- Material and travel costs

Developing objectives

- Training objectives - Desired trainee attitudinal & subjective evaluations of training
- Trainee reaction objectives-Objective set for how trainees should feel about the training and learning environment
- Learning objectives -Types of behaviour that demonstrate the learning
- Transfer of training objectives -Job Behaviour that affected by the training
- Organizational objectives-Organizational outcomes that will be affected by transfer of learning to the job & satisfaction of organizational objectives

How we identify objectives?

- Which performance deficiencies to be addressed
- Which are the needs to be learned in order to change job behaviour so that performance deficiencies are reduced

Components of objectives

- **Desired outcome**
  - What should be expected to occur
  - Trainee will be able to do at the end of training
- **Conditions**
  - Under what condition is the outcome
  - Condition under which the behaviour must occur
- **Standards**
  - What criteria signify that the outcome is acceptable
  - Criteria for success
  - Accuracy quality and speed

Learning objectives: Attitude

- Whether the trainee will be able to apply the theories of motivation to different situations
- Whether the trainee will be able to recognize and identify different personalities, and know how to motivate them
- Whether the trainee will be able to understand what is necessary to have an effective team
- Whether the trainee will be able to have knowledge of three types of active listening and be able to use the appropriate one in a particular situation
- Will be able to say not boss and peers when asked to do extra work.

Use of training objectives:

HRD Against arguments

- Waste valuable time
- No practical in today's world
- Unrealistic for management training and other soft areas of training
- Move focus from other areas
- Inhibit flexibility

Use of training (learning) objectives: HRD Pro-arguments

1. Trainee
2. Designer
3. Trainer
4. Evaluator of training

Use of training (learning) objectives:

1. Trainee
   - They reduce the anxiety
   - Focus on attention
   - Increase the likelihood that they will be successful in training
2. Designer
   - Guide the trainer kind of programme to be scheduled and preparation can be made based on outcome
3. Trainer
   - Can facilitate the learning process more effectively
   - Allow the trainer to evaluate trainees progressing
   - Make possible adjustment
4. Evaluator of training
   - Evaluation will be easier when objectives are used
   - The expected behaviour at the end of training

Facilitation of Learning

Focus on Trainee

- Trainees readiness for training
- Some employee want higher skills
- While some want minimum skills (job analysis)
- Individual differences in background/trait affects learning preferences
- More than job analysis individual analysis required
- Other wise it will boring to people who want it and who doesn't want it.

Motivation of the trainee

- If motivation is lacking no training is going to happen
- Training provides motivation and satisfaction

Expectation towards training

- Those with Positive expectations are more successful and motivated
- *"Even if I fail, this training will be a valuable experience"*
- *"I will get more from this training than most people"*
- *"I have a better chance of passing this training than most leaders"*
- *"If I have trouble during training, I will try harder"*

Expectancy theory implications

Positive outcomes lead to performance

- Promotion
- Better at job
- Less job stress
- Better team work
- Fewer grievances

Implication from conditioning

- Classical conditioning
- Stimuli Response
- Pleasant emotional responses are conditioned to situation
- Pleasant stimulus situations to be developed to create comfortable and pleasurable response from training
- Operant conditioning
- Response Stimuli
- Trainees should be reinforced for their efforts to learn regardless of the degree of success
- Consequent oriented behaviour
- More positive reinforcement training approach than negative reinforcement

- Trainees have a negative attitude towards role pays. If role plays are included, positive reinforcement strategies to be incorporated.

Implication from goal setting

Belief:

- Specific goals direct the individuals energy and attention toward meeting the goal.
- A number of conditions related to goal setting affect performance
- *Individual who has given challenging goal perform better than and soft goal*
- *Goals must be matched with the ability of individuals*
- *Individual needs to accept the goal that is set*
- *Feed back on desired goal to be provided*

Social Learning Theory

Paying Attention

- The first step in motivating employees and setting their expectations are to notify them that they will be participating in the training
- This indicates the training objectives
- Reiterating the objectives helps to keep the focus on the desired outcomes and attention on the important training activities
- The trainees must accept the objectives
- The trainer should ask the trainees how the training helps to resolve the job situations
- It focus attention and commitment of trainees

Cognitive Resource Allocation Theory (How Brain is used)

- How well you pay attention determines how much you learn.
- How well you pay attention determines how well you perform.
- The greater your intelligence, the more you pay attention.
- If you're motivated, you pay attention.

Retention - Four Stages

- Activation of memory
- Symbolic coding

- Cognitive organization
- Symbolic Rehearsal and cues for retrieval

Activation of memory

- Information to be converted into long term memory.
- Before new learning starts the connection between old and new to be established.
- It helps to recall relevant supportive learning.
- Through role plays on different situations different roles on decision making can be recalled from the prior learning.

Symbolic Coding and Cognitive Organization

- Once appropriate prior learning is recalled the trainee is ready to encode the new information.
- Encoding can also enhance through the use of images in addition to be coded as verbal proposition.
- Symbolic Coding incorporates both verbal propositions and images.
- Symbolic Coding and Cognitive Organization.
- Cognitive organization is intimately tied to symbolic coding.
- The way information is organized during training and the prior learning that supports learning the new information the way the new information is organized into cognitive structure.
- Symbolic Rehearsal and cues for retrieval
    - *Symbolic rehearsal and reproduction are types of practice.*
    - *Symbolic rehearsal is practicing symbolically as when the trainees ask the trainees to imagine the hypothetical situation and discuss how they would behave.*

Behavioural reproduction

- Is the transformation of the learning into actual behaviour
- Pilot training provides a clear example of difference between these two types of practices
- When a sufficient amount of learning occurs the trainees starts demonstration of the same.

Strategic knowledge

- Declarative knowledge
- Forming a mental picture of the task
- Knowledge compilation
- Integrating knowledge and motor skills
- Procedural knowledge
- Ability to perform task automatically, paying little attention to it.

Step 1

- Declarative knowledge (what) is presented (traditional training)
- Workers are told that the materials are designed to teach them to read and interpret quality control charts used through out their organization
- (Strategic knowledge is same as that of traditional training)

Step 2

Procedural knowledge (how) is to be presented

- Workers are assisted in recalling specific math skills. Then stimulus materials and information required to master the task are presented.
- (Strategic knowledge is same as that of traditional training)

Step 3

- Workers practice using the charts and interpreting the results. Then stimulus materials and information required to master the task are presented.
- (Strategic knowledge is same as that of traditional training)

Step 4

- Workers participate using the charts and interpreting the results
- Strategic knowledge training : Workers provide opportunity for rehearsal and reinforcement of both conditional and procedural)

Step 5

- Workers are given feedback
- Strategic knowledge training (feedback) same as that of traditional.

Facilitation of Transfer

Transfer of training

- Positive transfer
    - *A higher level of job performance*
- Zero transfer
    - *No change in job performance*
- Negative transfer
    - *A lower level of job transfer.*

Training Design Issues

- Conditions of practice
- Retention of what is learned

Conditions of Practice

Over learning

- Continuous practice far beyond the point at which they perform the task successfully. The more the task is learned greater the retention.

Task sequencing

- Each component task should be arranged in the proper sequence
- Some are serial tasks
- Some can be done in parallel

Knowledge of results (feedback)

- It tells the trainee whether their response is correct
- It makes the learning more interesting, encouraging trainees to continue
- It leads to specific goals for maintaining or improving performance.

Maximizing Transfer

- Identical elements
- Training design identical to real work environment, learning will be higher

Physical fidelity

- Physical accuracy, exactness

Psychological fidelity

- Mental closeness/detachment

Identical Elements

- The closer the training is to the job, the easier it is to achieve transfer
- Direct relationship to the job
- Example: Customer service and angry customers
- Role playing, business games, etc.

Physical Fidelity

- Same physically
- Same procedurally
- Example: Flight and submarine simulators
- Trainee experiences same stresses and conditions as he/she is being trained for
- Example: MS Flight Simulator

Support in Work Environment

- Transfer of training into workplace is supported
- A continuous learning environment
- Supervisors support and help develop training
- Training leads to promotion/better pay
- Trainee has opportunity to perform

Facilitation of transfer of learning

- Supervisory support
- Peer support
- Trainer support
- Reward system
- Organizational climate
- Organizational culture

Gagne's Theory of Instruction

- Verbal information
- Intellectual skills

- Cognitive strategies
- Motor skills
- Attitudes

ALL ARE LEARNED IN DIFFERENT WAYS

Gagne's Instructional Events

- Gain attention
- Ask questions of trainees to initiate interest in topic of feedback
- State the learning objective
- Show objectives and discuss
- Stimulate recall of earlier lessons
- Get trainees to verbalize things that they learned
- Present new material
- Specific and general information
- Provide learning guidance
- Provide Multiple examples
- Elicit performance
- Test the trainees cognitive level after training toward performance
- Provide feedback
- Get the feed back about the effectiveness about the training
- Assess performance
- Conduct a quiz to recall all the rules for effective feedback.
- Enhance retention and training transfer
- Trainees will back to learn the behavioural component of training in a week. Facilitate retention

Summary

Without learning, there would be no field of human resource development. To increase learning, we must consider:

- Trainee characteristics/individual differences
- Training design issues
- Retention and transfer of training issues

Training and HRD Process Model

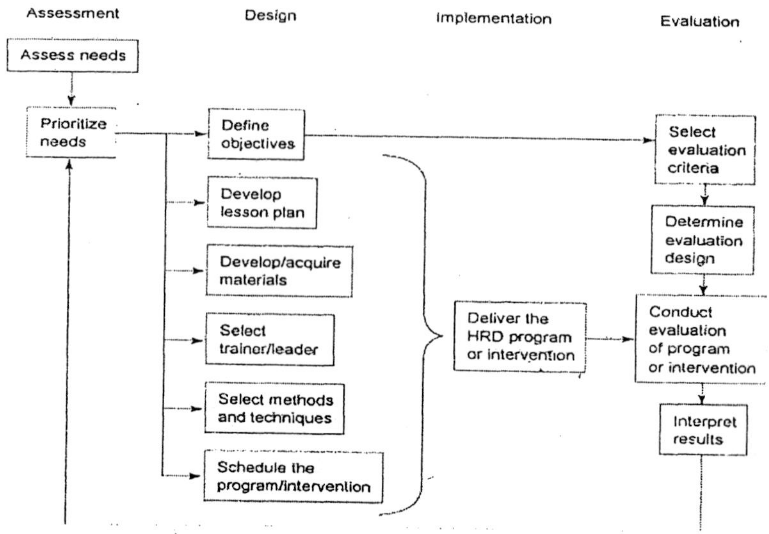

A Framework for the HRD Process

HRD efforts should use the following four phases (or stages):

- Needs assessment
- Design
- Implementation
- Evaluation

Training & HRD Process Model - Needs Assessment Phase

- Establishing HRD priorities
- Defining specific training and objectives
- Establishing evaluation criteria

Needs Assessment Phase

- Purpose - Guides entire training process -Instructional objectives, training design and evaluation all stem directly from the needs assessment
- Should be a continual process
- Central for determining if problem is a training problem or related to other issues such as poor selection, low motivation, etc.

- Several components - Organization analysis, Requirements analysis, Task analysis and Person analysis, Organizational Analysis
- Purpose - Determine where in the organization training should be conducted and could be conducted concerned with system wide components of an organization that may impact training program

Organizational Analysis

- Organizational goals
- Training needs to be congruent with organization's goals
- Without consideration, training may be working at cross-purposes to the organization
- Problem: goals often not stated
- Real goals not same a stated goals
- Training may miss mark b/c no thought to philosophy and culture
- Training may focus on skills not valued by org, even if needed for the job
- Organizational Training Climate
- Conflicts
- Trainer might get stuck between political wars and conflicting expectations
- Stated purpose not same as real expectations
- Top management support, lower levels don't care
- Overall resistance to change

External Constraints on Training

- Need to consider legal, social, economic and political factors
- Legal issues: Fair Employment Legislation says training must be accessible to minorities; must avoid adverse impact or validate training
- Insure required resources: money, materials and staff

Training and Management Responsibilities

- Act as change Agent
- Planning and Organizing change implementation

- Effective control over training
- Relate training with ROI
- Financial and operational performance improvement

Structure of Training Organization

Training as continuous improvement – Problem solving process

- Identifying organizations problems
- Determining the cause of the problem
- Identifying, implementing the best solutions
- Evaluating the effectiveness of solution
- Implementing the feedback
- Next focus of action

Why conduct a training need analysis?

- Align the training activities with the strategic plan
- Whether the deficiency can be corrected through training
- Making provision of the bench mark knowledge skill and attitude
- Careful analysis of the benchmarking competencies
- Training time, money and the resources spend wisely
- Determine the bench mark for evaluation of training
- Increase the motivation of participants
- Relevance of training
- Two approaches
    - *Proactive training and reactive training*
    - Proactive – anticipated performance (strategic plan)
    - Reactive – perceived performance problem (discrepancy)
- Where performance problem exists
- Where skill gap exists

Where the performance Discrepancy?

- Organizational goals and objectives and budgets
- Labour inventory
- Analysis of efficiency Indexes

- Cost of labour
- Cost of materials
- Quality of product
- Equipment utilization
- Cost of distribution
- Waste
- Downtime
- Late delivers
- Repairs
- Organizational climate index
- Labour management data, strikes, lockouts etc.
- Grievances
- Turnover
- Absenteeism
- Suggestions
- Productivity
- Accidents
- Short term sickness
- Observation of employee behaviour
- Attitude surveys
- Changes in the system or sub system
- Management requests or management interrogation
- Exit interviews
- MBO or work planning and review systems

Effective training practices involve the use of an *instructional systems design process.* The instructional systems design process begins by conducting a *needs assessment.*

Before choosing a training method, it is important to determine:

- what type of training is necessary, and
- whether trainees are willing to learn

Needs Assessment

- Refers to the process used to determine whether training is necessary because needs assessment is the first step in the instructional design process:
- If it is poorly conducted, training will not achieve the outcomes or financial benefits the company expects
    - Causes and Outcomes of Needs Assessment

Organizational Analysis – involves determining:

- the appropriateness of training, given the business strategy
- resources available for training
- support by managers and peers for training

Task Analysis – involves:

- identifying the important tasks and knowledge, skill, and behaviors that need to be emphasized in training for employees to complete their tasks

Person Analysis – involves:

- determining whether performance deficiencies result from a lack of knowledge, skill, or ability (a training issue) or from a motivational or work design problem
- identifying who needs training
- determining employees' readiness for training

Expected performance – Actual performance = Performance discrepancy

Readiness for training refers to whether:

- Employees have the personal characteristics necessary to learn program content and apply it on the job.
- The work environment will facilitate learning and not interfere with performance.

Factors that influence employee performance and learning

Person Characteristics

- Ability and skill
- Attitudes and motivation

Input

- Understand need to perform
- Necessary resources (equipment, etc.)
- Interference from other job demands
- Opportunity to perform

Output

- Standard to judge successful performers

Consequences

- Positive consequences/incentives to perform
- Few negative consequences to perform

Feedback

- Frequent and specific feedback about how the job is performed

Person Analysis: ***Self-Efficacy***

Self-efficacy - the employees believe that they can successfully perform their job or learn the content of the training program

- The *job environment* can be threatening to many employees who may not have been successful in the past
- The *training environment* can also be threatening to people who have not received training or formal education for some length of time

Employees' self-efficacy level can be increased by:

- Letting employees know that the purpose of the training is to try to improve performance rather than to identify areas in which employees are incompetent
- Providing as much information as possible about the training program and purpose of training prior to the actual training
- Showing employees the training success of their peers who are now in similar jobs
- Providing employees with feedback that learning is under their control and they have the ability and the responsibility to overcome any learning difficulties they experience in the program

To ensure that the work environment enhances trainees' motivation to learn:

- Provide materials, time, job-related information, and other work aids necessary for employees to use new skills or behavior before participating in training programs
- Speak positively about the company's training programs to employees
- Let employees know they are doing a good job when they are using training content in their work
- Encourage work-group members to involve each other in trying to use new skills on the job by soliciting feedback and sharing training experiences and situations in which training content was helpful
- Provide employees with time and opportunities to practice and apply new skills or behaviors to their work

To determine if training is the best solution, assess whether:

- The performance problem is important and has the potential to cost the company a significant amount of money from lost productivity or customers
- Employees do not know how to perform effectively
- Perhaps they received little or no previous training or the training was ineffective
- Employees cannot demonstrate the correct knowledge or behavior
- Employees were trained but they infrequently or never used the training content on the job
- Performance expectations are clear (input) and there are no obstacles to performance such as faulty tools or equipment
- There are positive consequences for good performance, while poor performance is not rewarded
- Employees receive timely, relevant, accurate, constructive, and specific feedback about their performance (a feedback issue)
- Other solutions such as job redesign or transferring employees to other jobs are too expensive or unrealistic

Person Analysis: ***Is training the best solution?***

- If employees lack the knowledge and skill to perform and the other factors are satisfactory, training is needed
- If employees have the knowledge and skill to perform but input, output, consequences, or feedback are inadequate, training may not be the best solution

Task Analysis

- Task analysis results in a description of work activities, including tasks performed by the employee and the knowledge, skills, and abilities required to complete the tasks
- Should only be undertaken after you have determined from the *organizational analysis* that the company wants to devote time and money for training

Data sources for task analysis

- Job description
- Job specification
- Performance standards
- Perform the job
- Observe job-work sampling
- Review of literature concerning job
    - In professional journals
    - In practitioner journals Form other industries
- Ask questions about the job
    - Of the job holder
    - Of the job supervisor

Steps in a Task Analysis

Select the job(s) to be analyzed

- Work oriented approach - general
- Task oriented approach – specific responsibilities

- Develop a preliminary list of tasks performed by the job
- List the knowledge related o the task.

- Validate or confirm the preliminary list of tasks
- Identify the knowledge, skills, or abilities necessary to successfully perform each task
- How important the task?

What you should get from job analysis

- Knowledge
- Skill
- Attitude
- Expected performance

Key Points to Remember When Conducting a Task Analysis

- Task analysis should identify both what employees are *actually doing* and what they *should be doing* on the job
- Task analysis begins by breaking the job into duties and tasks
- Use more than two methods for collecting task information to increase the validity of the analysis

For task analysis to be useful, information needs to be collected from subject matter experts (SMEs)

SMEs include:

- Job incumbents
- Managers
- Employees familiar with the job
    - In deciding how to evaluate tasks, the focus should be on *tasks necessary to accomplish the company's goals and objectives*
- These may not be the tasks that are the most difficult or take the most time

Competency

- A competency refers to areas of personal capability that enable employees to successfully perform their jobs by achieving outcomes or successfully performing tasks
    - A competency can be knowledge, skills, attitudes, values, or personal characteristics

Why competency?

- They are more general in nature
- They show a longer term fit.
- They include knowledge, skills feelings and motivation
- They tie into corporate goals.

Competency Model

- A competency model identifies the competencies necessary for each job as well as the knowledge, skills, behavior, and personality characteristics underlying each competency

Competency models are useful for training and development in several ways:

- They identify behaviors needed for effective job performance
- They provide a tool for determining what skills are needed to meet today's needs as well as the company's future skill needs
- They help determine what skills are needed at different career points

Competency models are useful for training and development in several ways:

- They provide a framework for ongoing coaching and feedback to develop employees for current and future roles
- They create a "roadmap" for identifying and developing employees who may be candidates for managerial positions

Outcome of Needs Assessment

Understand non-training needs

- Job aids
- Practice

Changing the job itself

- This information is used to develop training objectives, design training, and evaluate its effectiveness
- Pitfalls

Scope of Needs Assessment

- Time constraints can limit the length and detail obtained from needs assessment
- The scope of the needs assessment depends on the size of the potential *"pressure point"*
- You will be able to anticipate training needs if you are attuned to the:
  - business problems
  - technological developments
  - other issues facing the organization

SUMMARY

Training is referred to as a method to give the new entrant or an existing employee the skills, knowledge and attitude needed to perform the job. Training must be based on scientific approach and quality training material to meet objective number one. The training duration should be as short as possible and resources used efficiently for meeting objective required.

The *goal of training* is for employees to Master the knowledge, skill, and behaviors emphasized in training programs, and apply them to their day-to-day activities. Thus training plays a vital role in Human Resource Development.

UNIT 4

HUMAN RESOURCE DEVELOPMENT AND ORGANIZATION EFFECTIVENESS

INTRODUCTION

Organizational effectiveness is the concept of how *effective* an organization is achieving the *outcomes* the organization intends to produce. The idea of organizational effectiveness is especially important for *non-profit organizations* as most people who donate money to non-profit organizations and charities are interested in knowing whether the organization is effective in accomplishing its goals.

"Organizational effectiveness is the degree to which the organization achieves a stated goal. It means the organization succeeds in accomplishing what it tries to do. Organizational effectiveness means providing a product or service that customers value."

An organization's effectiveness is also dependent on its communicative competence and ethics. The relationship between these three are simultaneous. Ethics is a foundation found within organizational effectiveness. An organization must exemplify respect, honesty, integrity and equity to allow communicative competence with the participating members. Along with ethics and communicative competence, members in that particular group can finally achieve their intended goals.

Foundations and other sources of *grants* and other types of funds are interested in organizational effectiveness of those people who seek funds from the foundations. Foundations always have more requests for funds or funding *proposals* and treat funding as an *investment* using the same care as a *venture capitalist* would in picking a company in which to invest.

How can the effectiveness of an organization be measured? Organizational effectiveness is an abstract concept and is basically impossible to measure. Instead of measuring organizational effectiveness, the organization determines proxy measures which will be used to represent effectiveness. Proxy measures used may include such things as number of people served, types and sizes of population segments served, and the demand within those segments for the services the organization supplies.

For instance, a non-profit organization which supplies meals to *house bound* people may collect statistics such as the number of meals cooked and served, the number of *volunteers* delivering meals, the turnover and retention rates of volunteers, the *demographics* of the people served, the turnover and retention of consumers, the number of requests for meals turned down due to lack of capacity (amount of food, capacity of meal preparation facilities, and number of delivery volunteers), and amount of wastage. Since the organization has as its goal the preparation of meals and the delivery of those meals to house bound people, it measures its organizational effectiveness by trying to determine what actual activities the people in the organization do in order to generate the outcomes the organization wants to create.

Activities such as *fund raising* or volunteer training are important because they provide the support needed for the organization to deliver its services but they are not the outcomes per se. These other activities are overhead activities which assist the organization in achieving its desired outcomes.

To be effective and achieve its goals, an organization must successfully respond to environmental factors. Various models of determining organizational effectiveness exist because organizations face different environments, they produce different products, their organizational members are made up of different kinds of people, and the organizations are at different stages of development. Each model is most useful to an organization having a particular combination of these environmental and organizational attributes.

- Two different underlying dimensions may be considered to develop models of organizational effectiveness. The first is the organization's internal versus external focus. The second dimension is the organization's emphasis on flexibility versus control. Flexibility allows faster change, whereas control allows a firmer grasp on current operations. When these two dimensions are drawn at right angles to each other, the first four models of organizational effectiveness can be plotted. They are the rational goal, open system, internal process, and human relations models.

- According to the **rational goal model** of effectiveness, an organization is effective to the extent that it accomplishes its stated goals. For example, the formal goals of the Toronto Blue Jays are to win their division, the American League pennant, and the World Series.
- With an **open system model** an organization is effective to the degree that it acquires inputs from its environment and has outputs accepted by its environment. The University of Alberta follows this model when it is concerned about the quality and number of students applying for admission and what jobs they receive on graduation.
- The **internal process model** focuses on the effectiveness of the internal transformation process. When Hamilton's Stelco Inc. examines its steel-making methods to determine price and quality competitiveness, it is focusing on its internal processes.
- The **human relations model** focuses on the development of the organization's personnel. Marlin Travel sends its agents on familiarization trips to expand their knowledge of specific hotels, cruises, and destinations.
- The **competing values model** requires that an organization scrutinize the balance among the above four effectiveness models. In this model there are three sets of competing values. The first is the tension between internal versus external focus. The more the organization focuses on one, the less it can concentrate on the other. For example Apple Computer has focused externally on its customers and making computers that are intuitive and easy to use. The computer chip maker Intel has had a more internal focus on how to make faster and more

powerful central processing units at a low price. The second set of values in competition is flexibility versus control. Flexibility allows quick response to changing conditions and values innovation. Control values the opposite. Stability and predictability mean that routine activities are performed well but change is more difficult. The third set of competing values is the relative concern with the feelings, needs, and development of the people making up the organization versus the organization and its requirement to accomplish its tasks.

- A private hospital, for example, is concerned with how patients are treated and the success rate of surgeries (the rational goal model). It is also interested in how hospital procedures are performed (the internal process model) and with the skills and abilities of hospital staff (the human relations model). Finally, because it is a private hospital and must make a profit to survive, it needs to take into account how many and what kinds of patients are admitted (the open system model). The hospital must balance the three sets of competing values in order to be effective.
- With the **strategic constituencies model** an organization would aim to at least minimally satisfy the most important constituents (or stakeholders) in its environment. The owner of an A&W franchise must satisfy the customers and A&W head office management. Customers care about the quality and price of the food as well as the speed and friendliness of service. Head office cares about these issues along with financial reporting, product promotions, and the store's relationship with its community.
- An organization seeking **legitimacy** survives by acting in a manner seen by other organizations as legitimate. An example would be producing a business plan and projected income statement in order to obtain a bank loan.
- The organization adopting the **fault-driven model** of effectiveness seeks to eliminate traces of ineffectiveness in its internal functioning. The National Aeronautics and Space Administration (NASA) in the United States is a good example.

Its systems are designed with backups to be reliable even if some components fail.

- Finally, the organization as a **high performing system** compares itself to other similar organizations. The Vancouver Symphony Orchestra can measure ticket sales and customer satisfaction with performances. But to determine the quality of the orchestra itself, comparison is made to other orchestras in the world. Effectiveness is seen as the degree to which that comparison is positive. One method used by high performers to make such comparisons is to examine industry rankings. An example is the Maclean's magazine ratings of Canadian universities.

1. The most important aspects of research management for organizational effectiveness as perceived by the scientists are "management of human resources", "resource mobilization", "infrastructure development", and "research planning, project development and implementation".
2. The most important skills required to be a successful research manager are "managing people at work", "administration" and "supervision and monitoring".
3. The important changes need to be brought into management practices are "humanizing the environment in organizations", "professional management approach" and "visibility with outside agencies".
4. The most usual impediments to change are the "resistance from junior cadre scientists", "negative attitude of staff", "personal egos of senior colleagues" and "frequent changes in the way of management".
5. The broad areas for HRD interventions for research managers are "managing the research", "managing the people", "managing the resources" and "information and communication technology".
6. Based on the brainstorming sessions the most salient recommendations are classified under five major areas such as "*institutional autonomy, research management, accountability, personnel policies and HRD for women*". The foremost recommendations are to provide more delegation of powers at all levels to decentralize the function of management,

ICAR to develop its own administrative and financial rules to avail full functional autonomy, introduce project based budgeting and accountability through five yearly assessment target in research output, reduce the administrative procedures and channels, objective assessment of scientists and staff annually, introduce contract system of appointments for all cadres, change the system of interviews at ASRB, restore the old concept of ARS, provide welfare facilities for women.

7. On the issue of management training opportunities, introduce foundation courses for all categories of staff. Scientists of SAUs may be encouraged to avail management training opportunities at NAARM, NAARM to introduce foundation courses in educational technology, distance training options may be explored and the senior level management programmes at NAARM may also include RMPs and Heads from SAUs.
8. The personality type analysis of scientists of NARS reveals that there is need for training in personality development on the lines of neuro linguistic programmes (NLP), need for enhancing creativity among the rank and file of scientists and academicians, aptitude tests may be introduced at the entry level of scientists and introduce personality development in course curricula of UG and PG programmes.
9. The institutional survey of NARS stations and centers indicates that the manpower strength may be filled to the sanctioned cadre strength; there is need for enhancing ICT facilities, living conditions and other welfare measures, especially, in SAUs. E-mail and Internet connectivity in the stations of SAUs need a lot of overall improvement for effective use.
10. A comprehensive quantitative analysis on the HRD requirements of administrative and finance functionaries of ICAR was carried out and the most salient findings and recommendations are as follows:
    - Compulsory training at the entry level for all staff and refresher courses once in three years.
    - Officers and staff may be encouraged to attend job-related seminars and conferences to develop their perspectives.

- Need Evaluation Factors (NEF) for a variety of office functions were statistically calculated based on functional requirement, difficulties encountered, supervisors' choice of training and choice of Heads of Office. Accordingly, based on the NEF values obtained the training areas were classified on *Compulsory, Vital, Essential and Desirable* for the administrative and finance functionaries of ICAR.
- The compulsory areas for training include computer applications, salary, wages and claims administration, purchases and materials management.
- Vital areas of training include vigilance and disciplinary procedures, training and development, work-study, quality control of office work, agricultural research management, leadership, planning and execution of work, office communication and record keeping and public relations and networking.
- Five yearly assessments may be introduced for administrative and finance functionaries on the lines of the system followed for technical staff.
- Follow up plan of action for HRD interventions for administrative and finance functionaries have been suggested.

ORGANIZATIONAL LIFE CYCLE

- What makes an organization effective varies with its stage of development. As organizations pass through common stages throughout their life cycle their structure changes, their basis of growth changes, and their goals change. It should be remembered that organizations may not grow continuously but may remain at one stage of development for long periods.
- Most organizations are in operation for significantly fewer years than the average person lives. We know that failure is very common with new organizations. Restaurants, for example, are known to have high rates of startups and closures. This tendency is called the liability of newness. Older organizations die, too, though we often feel a sense of shock when we read of a well-

established company that closes its doors. A recent example is Eaton's.

- The first stage of an organization's development is its birth. Here growth is through creativity, the goal is survival, and the structure is non-bureaucratic. The organization's founder is often ruling the organization and does not rely on formalized rules and relationships. Predictable crises are encountered by growing organizations. The first crisis is that of leadership. Will the transition be made from being managed by the organization's founder to being managed by professional managers?
- The next stage of development is the organization's youth. Growth now is by direction, as professional managers brought into the company start to impose organizational rules and bureaucracy. The goal is growth and management aims to provide a sense of mission to members of the organization. The crisis faced at this stage is that senior managers may not wish to relinquish control to more junior managers by delegating tasks and authority to them.
- At the organization's mid-life, growth is through delegation and coordination, the goal is efficiency, and the structure becomes more bureaucratic and departmentalized. To be able to change from a red-tape bureaucracy to a collaborative-team-oriented organization is the crisis that will eventually arise. At maturity this collaboration will be achieved. The crisis at this stage is to avoid becoming stagnant and enduring a slow decline and eventual death. Instead, the organization must continually renew itself. In the final stage of decline and death some organizations cannot change because their management becomes a roadblock to change. Also, the organization's current structure can become a constraint on necessary change.

Organization Structure

- The founder of an organization has to make a series of decisions about what business to be in, what the organization's goals and objectives are, what work has to be performed to attain those goals, how the work will be divided and coordinated, and who will do the work. These decisions may be interdependent if the organization is small. Making one decision will affect others. For example, the skills and abilities of the particular people hired into the organization will then affect decisions about what the organization can do and how it will do it.

- A small organization, for example a shoe store, would have a simple structure. Here everyone, including the managers, is involved in selling. Some specialized functions, such as accounting and advertising, may be contracted out to a bookkeeper and an advertising agency. A small travel agency would also have a simple structure. It could consist of only two divisions, one with two sales agents working exclusively with corporate clients and the other with two agents selling personal holidays to the general public. The manager (who may also be the owner) would sell travel packages to corporate and holiday clients, hire and train staff, pay the bills, and try to build agency sales by finding new corporate and holiday clients.

Measures of Structure

Structure concerns more than the division of labour or the boxes on the organization chart. It is also about the reporting relationships between organizational members. These are the lines connecting the boxes, rules and regulations about how the work is performed, and whether organizational decisions are made at the top of the organization or lower down. In order to compare one organization's structure with that of another or to study the effects of structure on organizational performance, we need to have consistent ways to measure structure. Three important structure measures are complexity, formalization, and centralization.

Complexity refers to the number of separate parts in an organization's structure. The more tasks are divided among individuals and specialized, the more the organization is horizontally complex. As the vertical chain of command lengthens, more organizational layers are inserted between top management and production workers. The organization becomes more vertically complex. Vertical complexity is often also called the tallness of the organization. Organizations today are tending to move towards flatter organizations by eliminating whole levels of middle management. This downsizing increases the number of people supervised. Therefore the span of control increases for the managers that remain.

Formalization refers to the extent to which job activity is defined and controlled by rules. The more rules there are about how to do the work and how decisions are made, the more an organization is formalized. Police departments are often very formalized as the activities of officers are strictly controlled by rules that cover almost every situation that may arise. A campus radio station, on the other hand, may be much less formal, having only a few rules governing the broadcasting behaviour of station members.

Centralization concerns where in the organization decisions are made. When decision-making is reserved for top management, vertical centralization is high. Vertical centralization is low when lower-level employees in the hierarchy are given decision-making authority. Horizontal decentralization occurs when workers in many different organizational units are allowed to make decisions without referring to a more central authority.

These structural measures of complexity, centralization, and formalization may be combined into the two broad and descriptive categories of mechanistic and organic.

Mechanistic organizations were so named because they can be seen to operate as machines. They are characterized by highly specialized tasks that tend to be rigidly defined, have hierarchical authority and control, and communications that primarily take the form of instructions and decisions issued by superiors to subordinates. Communication is mostly vertical from the top down. Further, loyalty to the organization and obedience to superiors is a condition of membership. Mechanistic organizations tend to be complex, formalized, and centralized. An automobile factory that uses a production line technology is a good example of an organization with a mechanistic structure.

Organic organizations act more as living things. They have tasks that are more interdependent and that are continually adjusted and redefined through interaction with organizational members. An advertising agency such as Saatchi & Saatchi needs to be flexible in dealing with customers and in creating concepts for television commercials and print advertisements. In an organic organization, control depends less on formal job position and more on expertise relevant to the particular problem being considered. Communication is both vertical (up and down the hierarchy) and horizontal (across different departments of the organization) depending on where the needed information resides. These communications primarily take the form of information and advice. Commitment in the organic organization is to the organization's tasks and goals. Members accept general responsibility for task accomplishment beyond their individual role definition. That is, they do not stick to a job description as a definition of the work they will do. Organic organizations tend to be simple, low in formalization, and decentralized. They adapt to and create change in their environments.

Bureaucratic theory makes the assumption that people are rational and can work within the rules. These guide behaviour, meaning that conflict would be avoided. Weber provides guidelines for how to structure an organization. This is the ideal type bureaucracy, as it should work. Non-rational behaviour and conflict between individuals were not anticipated. We now know that non-rationality and conflict are present in bureaucratic structures.

Woodward and her colleagues found that organizations were more effective when their technology matched the organization's structure. Specifically, for small batch production, an organic structure was best because the production of custom items requires a good deal of informal communication and adaptation. Organizations using a mass production technology were more effective when using a mechanistic structure. The reason was that control over a complex and repetitive process could be effectively exerted by rules and regulations. When a continuous process technology was used, Woodward found that an organic structure was more effective. In this case highly trained technicians monitored machines producing the organization's output and needed to communicate freely about the production process and any irregularities that were noticed.

Organizational Effectiveness, within the Office of Human Resources, serves as a gateway to training, development, and consulting resources that build organizational capacity, increase individual capabilities, and promote a culture of excellence through strong leadership. The division collaborates with institutional stakeholders to strategically and systemically address the University's mission and goals.

Organizational Effectiveness offers a variety of programs and services designed to build job skills and enhance professional development. We provide workshops, seminars, classes, and consulting services to over 14,000 U of M participants each year. Our facilitators are also available for customized, onsite sessions for colleges, departments, areas, or work units.

Areas of service include:

- Employee Career Services
- Organizational Development
- Leadership Development
- Personal & Professional Development
- Supervisory Training and Development
- Training Services

HRD EXPERIENCES OF ORGANISATIONS

HRD function has got a good deal of attention in the recent past and is continuing to get more. The instruments of HRD are many. The HRD instruments should lead to the generation of HRD processes like role clarity, performance planning, development climate, risk-taking, dynamism, etc. in employees. Such HRD process should result in more competent, satisfied and committed people that would make the organization grow by contributing their best to it. Such HRD outcomes influence the organizational effectiveness. A model explaining the linkages between HRD instruments, processes, outcomes and organizational effectiveness is presented. Experiences of seven public sector and seven private sector organizations (BEMK, BHEL, Bank of Baroda, Crompton Greaves, Jyoti, Indian Oil Corporation, L&T, L&T-ECC, SAIL, State Bank of India, State Bank of Patiala, Sundaram Fasteners, TVS Iyengar & Sons and Voltas) were analysed against this model, The analysis suggests that new HRD departments, performance appraisals, role analysis and OD exercises have been the most frequently used HRD instruments. Using external consultants as well as internal task forces consisting of line managers, company-wide education of line managers and top managements' participation in the change process are most commonly observed in these organizations. However, very little evidence is available about the impact of the HRD instruments in terms of developing a HRD culture and HRD outcomes. It is argued that in the absence of a demonstration of such a linkage HRD becomes a matter of philosophy and faith. HRD departments have a complex role to play as even theoretically the links between HRD and organizational effectiveness are not easily demonstrable. HRD departments and top management should recognize this and accordingly plan their future strategies.

HRD CLIMATE

'HRD climate' helps the employees to acquire traits that would enable them to execute their present or future expected roles and aids in developing their capabilities for Organizational Development. A person's behavior is the outcome of several factors or motives. Motivation is one of the important factors affecting human behavior.

With organisations achieving a HRD climate, a basic source of human motivation to perform higher, human wastage has been reduced. So, whereas personnel management (PM) regarded wages and salaries as the main source of motivation, Human Resource Management (HRM) regards creation of a congenial work climate (HRD climate), job challenges, creativity and opportunity for development as the motivating forces. In other words, PM has worked in a smaller world of activities than Human Resource Management (HRM), which is concerned with the total organisation.

The concept of **organizational climate** has been assessed by various authors, of which many of them published their own definition of organisational climate. For those interested in understanding organizational climate, it is important to make some distinctions. First, climate and culture are both important aspects of the overall context, environment or situation. Culture tends to be shared by all or most members of some social group; is something that older members usually try to pass on to younger members; shapes behavior and structures perceptions of the world. Cultures are often studied and understood at a national level, such as the American or French culture. Culture includes deeply held values, beliefs and assumptions, symbols, heroes and heroines, and rituals. Culture can be examined at an organizational level as well. The main distinction between organizational and national culture is that people can choose to join a place of work, but are usually born into a national culture.

Organizational cultures are generally deep and stable. Climate, on the other hand, is often defined as the recurring patterns of behavior, attitudes and feelings that characterize life in the organization (Isaksen & Ekvall, 2007). Although culture and climate are related, climate often proves easier to assess and change. At an individual level of analysis the concept is called individual psychological climate. These individual perceptions are often aggregated or collected for analysis and understanding at the team or group level, or the divisional, functional, or overall organizational level.

Organisational climate, however, proves to be hard to define. There are two especially intractable and related difficulties: how to define *climate* and how to measure it effectively on different levels of analysis. Furthermore there are several approaches to the concept of climate, of which two in particular have received substantial patronage: the *cognitive schema* approach and the *shared perception* approach.

The first approach regards the concept of climate as an individual perception and cognitive representation of the work environment. From this perspective climate assessments should be conducted at an individual level.

The second approach emphasizes the importance of shared perceptions as underpinning the notion of climate (Anderson, & West, 1998; Mathisen & Einarsen 2004). Reichers and Schneider (1990) define organisational climate as "the shared perception of the way things are around here" (p. 22). It is important to realize that from these two approaches, there is no "best" approach and they actually have a great deal of overlap.

Organisational Climate (sometimes known as Corporate Climate) is the process of quantifying the "culture" of an organisation.

Researchers Hart, Griffin, Wearing & Cooper (1996) have pursued the shared perception model of Organisational Climate. Their model identifies the variables which moderate an organisation's ability to mobilise its workforce in order to achieve business goals and maximise performance.

One of the major users of this model includes many departments of the Queensland State Government (Australia). These departments use this model of Climate to survey staff to identify and measure those aspects of a workplace which impact on: stress, morale, quality of worklife, well-being, employee engagement, absenteeism/ presenteeism, turnover and performance.

While an organisation and its leaders cannot remove every stressor in the daily life of its employees, Organisational Climate studies have identified a number of behaviours of leaders which have a significant impact on stress and morale. For instance, one Queensland state government employer, Queensland Transport has found that increasing managers' awareness of these behaviours has improved quality of work life employees and the ability of QT's to deliver its organisational goals.

Theories of Cognitive and Neuropsychology and Emotional Intelligence provide additional scientific rationale for why leaders should improve stress and morale in the workplace to achieve maximum performance. Climate surveys can provide concrete evidence of how this works in action.

Organisational Climate surveying enables the impact of HR strategies to be evaluated to create HR Return on Investment (HRROI) calculations. This data has been found to be highly effective in changing the perspective of people-based initiatives as being an "investment" rather than a "cost" and transforming HR into a "mission-critical strategic partner" from its perception of "personnel administration".

A number of studies by Dr. Dennis Rose and colleagues (2001, 2002, 2004) have found a very strong link between Organisational

Climate and employee reactions such as stress levels, absenteeism and commitment and participation. A study by Heidi Bushell (2007) has found that Hart, Griffin et al.'s (1996) Organisational Climate model accounts for at least 16% single-day sick leave and 10% separation rates in one organisation. Other studies support the links between organizational climate and many other factors such as employee retention, job satisfaction, well-being, and readiness for creativity, innovation and change. Hunter, Bedell and Mumford (2007) have reviewed numerous approaches to climate assessment for creativity. They found that those climate studies that were based on well-developed, standardized instruments produced far higher effect sizes than did studies that were based on locally developed measures.

PERFORMANCE APPRAISAL

Performance appraisal, also known as **employee appraisal**, is a method by which the *job performance* of an *employee* is evaluated (generally in terms of *quality*, *quantity*, *cost* and *time*). Performance appraisal is a part of *career development*.

Performance appraisals are regular reviews of employee performance within *organizations*.

Generally, the aims of a performance appraisal are to:

- Give feedback on performance to employees.
- Identify employee *training* needs.
- *Document* criteria used to allocate organizational *rewards*.
- Form a basis for personnel decisions: *salary* increases, *promotions*, *disciplinary actions*, etc.
- Provide the opportunity for organizational diagnosis and development.
- Facilitate communication between employee and administration
- Validate selection techniques and human resource policies to meet federal Equal Employment Opportunity requirements.

A common approach to assessing performance is to use a numerical or *scalar* rating system whereby managers are asked to score an individual against a number of *objectives*/attributes. In some companies, employees receive assessments from their *manager*, peers, subordinates and *customers* while also performing a self assessment. This is known as 360° appraisal, forms good communication patterns

The most popular methods that are being used as performance appraisal process are:

- *Management by objectives*
- *360 degree appraisal*
- *Behavioral Observation Scale*
- *Behaviorally Anchored Rating Scale*

Trait based systems, which rely on factors such as *integrity* and *conscientiousness*, are also commonly used by businesses. The scientific literature on the subject provides evidence that assessing employees on factors such as these should be avoided. The reasons for this are two-fold:

1. Because trait based systems are by definition based on *personality traits*, they make it difficult for a manager to provide feedback that can cause positive change in employee performance. This is caused by the fact that personality *dimensions* are for the most part *static*, and while an employee can change a specific *behavior* they cannot change their *personality*. For example, a person who lacks integrity may stop lying to a manager because they have been caught, but they still have low integrity and are likely to lie again when the threat of being caught is gone.
2. Trait based systems, because they are vague, are more easily influenced by *office politics*, causing them to be less reliable as a source of information on an employee's true performance. The vagueness of these instruments allows managers to fill them out based on who they want to/feel should get a raise, rather than basing scores on specific behaviors employees should/should not be engaging in. These systems are also more likely to leave a company open to *discrimination* claims because a manager can make *biased* decisions without having to back them up with specific behavioral information.

POTENTIAL APPRAISAL AND CAREER DEVELOPMENT

Employees aspire to grow and expect this growth to take place at frequent intervals. Achievement of organisational goal, increased productivity and fulfilment of corporate objectives can be possible only if the employees are feeling satisfaction and achievement. To achieve this there is a requirement for a well thought out system of career and succession planning in an organisation. In this backdrop, this unit deals with mechanisms of potential appraisals and ways and means employed by organizations such as assessment centres to provide growth opportunities to employees. Many companies, which carry out performance appraisal, also keep records on the potential of their employees for future promotion opportunities. The task of identifying potential for promotion cannot be easy for the appraising manager, since competence of a member of staff to perform well in the current job is not an automatic indicator of potential for promotion. Very often the first class salesman is promoted to become a mediocre sales manager, the excellent chief engineer is promoted to become a very poor engineering director, and the star football player struggles to be a football manager. Potential can be defined as 'a latent but unrealised ability'. There are many people who have the desire and potential to advance through the job they are in, wanting the opportunity to operate at a higher level of competence in the same type of work. The potential is the one that the appraiser should be able to identify and develop because of the knowledge of the job. This requires an in-depth study of the positions which may become vacant, looking carefully at the specific skills that the new position may demand and also taking into consideration the more subjective areas like 'qualities' required. These may be areas where the employee has not had a real opportunity to demonstrate the potential ability and there may be areas with which you, as the appraisers are not familiar.

PSYCHOLOGICAL STRATEGIES OF HRD – PRINCIPLES

Business organizations exist in a competitive environment with scarce resources. Controlling these resources (physical, organizational, information and human) that gives the company the competitive advantage. The goal of strategic management in an organization is to deploy and allocate resources in order to provide the management with a competitive advantage. It goes without saying that two out of three classes of resources (organizational and human) correlated with the human resource functions. Towards maximum effect, the HRM functions must be integrally involved in the company's strategic management process. Strategic management process first analyzes a company's competitive situation, develops its strategic goals and mission, it's external opportunities and threats, and its internal strength and weaknesses to generate alternatives. In his second phase, strategic management process determines a plan of actions and deployment of resources to achieve the pre-specified goals. This kind of strategic approach should be emphasized in human resources management. Strategic human resources management (SHRM) is the pattern of planned human resources deployments and activities intended to enable an organization to achieve its goals. Then we are addressing the question of the instruments that will make the odds of the competition in our favour.

Four levels of integration exist between the HR functions and the strategic management function:

- Administrative linkage: HR function's attention is focused on day-to-day activities
- One-way linkage: the firm develops the strategic plan and then informs the R.
- Two-way linkage: strategic planning team informs HR of the various strategies, HR analyze them and present the results to the team. After deciding, the strategic plan is passed to HR to implement.
- Integrative linkage: it is a dynamic process, based on continuing rather than sequential interaction, done by the HR executive who is a member of the senior management team.

Strategy formulation consists of five major components

- Mission is a statement of the organization's reason for being, customers served and their needs, and the technology used. Also presents the company's vision and values.
- Goals are what the firm hopes to achieve in the medium-to-long term future.

- External analysis examines the firm's operating environment to identify the strategic opportunities and threats.
- Internal analysis identifies the firm's strengths and weaknesses, focuses on the quantity and quality of resources available.
- Strategic choice is done after the Strengths Weaknesses Opportunities Threats (SWOT) analysis to define strategic alternatives, and then the choice is made among these alternatives. Mechanisms for integration the HR function into strategy formulation may help the strategic planning team to make the most effective strategic choice, since HR will implement it.

It is now time to execute the strategy formulated, indicating certain HR needs. HR function can be viewed as having six menus of HR practices from which companies can choose the ones that are most appropriate to implementing the strategy. While, all of the strategy types require competent people in a generic sense, each of the strategies also requires different types of employees with types of behaviours and attitudes. The emerging strategic role of the HR function requires that HR professionals in the future develop business, professional-technical, change management, and integration competencies. The following figure will illustrate the model of the strategic management process.

SUMMARY

Organizational effectiveness is the degree to which the organization achieves a stated goal. It means the organization succeeds in accomplishing what it tries to do. Organizational effectiveness means providing a product or service that customers value."

The most important aspects of research management for organizational effectiveness as perceived by the scientists are "management of human resources", "resource mobilization", "infrastructure development", and "research planning, project development and implementation".

HRD departments have a complex role to play as even theoretically the links between HRD and organizational effectiveness are not easily demonstrable. HRD departments and top management should recognize this and accordingly plan their future strategies. A **chief executive officer (CEO)** or **chief executive** is one of the highest-ranking *corporate officer* (*executive*) or *administrator* in charge of total *management*. An individual selected as President and CEO of a *corporation*, *company*, *organization*, or *agency*, reports to the *board of directors*. In internal communication and press releases, many companies capitalize the term and those of other high positions, even when they are not *proper nouns*.

'HRD climate' helps the employees to acquire traits that would enable them to execute their present or future expected roles and aids in developing their capabilities for Organizational Development. Organizational cultures are generally deep and stable. Climate, on the other hand, is often defined as the recurring patterns of behavior, attitudes and feelings that characterize life in the organization.

UNIT 5

ORGANIZATIONAL DEVELOPMENT IN HUMAN RESOURCE DEVELOPMENT

INTRODUCTION

The first HRD department in the Indian corporate sector was started in 1975 in Larsen and Toubro as per the recommendations of two consultants, Udai Pareek and T.V. Rao, from Indian Institute of Management, Ahmedabad. This was followed by State Bank if India and its associate banks. Two years later, one of the largest public sector companies in India, Bharat Earth Movers Limited, Bangalore, established its HRD department.

In the late seventies, there were hardly a dozen organizations with HRD departments. But by the eighties many had started establishing them. By mid eighties the importance of HRD had grown to such an extent that almost every second organization in India had established an HRD department. In the nineties almost every organization had an HRD department with the function being institutionalized.

The Pareek and Rao's Model envisaged the HRD function as consisting of 6 subsystems, viz.,

1. Development oriented performance appraisal
2. Potential appraisal
3. Training
4. Feedback and counselling
5. Career planning and development and
6. Organizational development.

All these 6 subsystems are linked to one another and a part of human resource system.

ORGANIZATIONAL DEVELOPMENT

Kurt Lewin (1898 - 1947) is widely recognized as the founding father of Organizational Development (OD), although he died before the concept became current in the mid-1950s. At the core of OD is the concept of *organization*, defined as two or more people working together toward one or more shared goals. Development in this context is the notion that an organization may become more effective over time at achieving its goals.

OD is a long range effort to improve organization's problem solving and renewal processes, particularly through more effective and collaborative management of organizational culture, often with the assistance of a change agent or catalyst and the use of the theory and technology of applied behavioral science.

Today's organizations operate in a rapidly changing environment. Consequently, one of the most important assets for an organization is the ability to manage change — and for people to remain healthy and authentic.

Definitions of OD

"Organization Development is the attempt to influence the members of an organization to expand their candidness with each other about their views of the organization and their experience in it, and to take greater responsibility for their own actions as organization members. The assumption behind OD is that when people pursue both of these objectives simultaneously, they are likely to discover new ways of working together that they experience as more effective for achieving their own and their shared (organizational) goals. And that when this does not happen, such activity helps them to understand why and to make meaningful choices about what to do in light of this understanding." —Neilsen

"Organization development is a system-wide application of behavioral science knowledge to the planned development and reinforcement of organizational strategies, structures, and processes for improving an organization's effectiveness." —Cummings and Worley

As defined by *Richard Beckhard*, "Organization development" (OD) is a planned, top-down, organization-wide effort to increase the organization's effectiveness and health. OD is achieved through interventions in the organization's "processes," using *behavioural science* knowledge.

According to *Warren Bennis*, "OD is a complex strategy intended to change the beliefs, attitudes, values, and structure of organizations so that they can better adapt to new technologies, markets, and challenges.

Warner Burke emphasizes that - "OD is not just *anything done to better an organization*; it is a particular kind of change process designed to bring about a particular kind of end result. OD involves organizational reflection, system improvement, planning, and self-analysis.

Organization Development is a body of knowledge and practice that enhances organizational performance and individual development, viewing the organization as a complex system of systems that exist within a larger system, each of which has its own attributes and degrees of alignment. OD interventions in these systems are inclusive methodologies and approaches to strategic planning, organization design, leadership development, change management, performance management, coaching, diversity, and work/life balance.

Organizational development is an ongoing, systematic process to implement effective change in an organization. Organizational development is known as both a field of applied behavioral science focused on understanding and managing organizational change and as a field of scientific study and inquiry. It is interdisciplinary in nature and draws on sociology, psychology, and theories of motivation, learning, and personality.

Organization development is a *contractual relationship* between a *change agent* and a *sponsoring organization* entered into for the purpose of *using applied behavioral science* in a *systems context* to *improve organizational performance* and the *capacity of the organization to improve itself.*

Contractual Relationship: Although neither the sponsoring *organization* nor the change agent can be sure at the outset of the exact nature of the problem or problems to be dealt with or how long the change agents' help will be needed, it is essential that some tentative agreement on these matters be reached. The sponsoring organization needs to know generally what the change agent's preliminary plan is, what its own commitments are in relation to personal commitments and responsibility for the program, and what the change agent's fee will be. The change agent must assure himself that the organization's, and particularly the top executives', commitment to change is strong enough to support the kind of *self-analysis* and personal involvement requisite to success of the program. Recognizing the uncertainties lying ahead on both sides, a termination agreement permitting either side to withdraw at any time is usually included.

Change Agent: A change agent in the sense used here is not a *technical expert* skilled in such functional areas as accounting, production, or finance. He is a behavioral scientist who knows how to get people in an organization involved in solving their own problems. His main strength is a comprehensive knowledge of human behavior, supported by a number of intervention techniques (to be discussed later). The change agent can be either external or internal to the organization. An internal change agent is usually a staff person who has expertise in the behavioral sciences and in the intervention technology of OD. Beckhard reports several cases in which line people have been trained in OD and have returned to their organizations to engage in successful change assignments. In the natural evolution of change mechanisms in organizations, this would seem to approach the ideal arrangement. Qualified change agents can be found on some university faculties, or they may be private consultants associated with such organizations as the National Training Laboratories Institute for Applied Behavioral Science (*Washington, D.C.*) or *University Associates* (*San Diego, California*), and similar organizations.

The change agent may be a staff or line member of the organization who is schooled in OD theory and technique. In such a case, the "contractual relationship" is an in-house agreement that should probably be explicit with respect to all of the conditions involved except the fee.

Sponsoring Organization: The initiative for OD programs comes from an organization that has a problem. This means that top management or someone authorized by top *management* is aware that a problem exists and has decided to seek help in solving it. There is a direct analogy here to the practice of psychotherapy: The *client* or *patient* must actively seek help in finding a solution to his problems. This indicates a willingness on the part of the client organization to accept help and assures the organization that management is actively concerned.

Applied Behavioral Science: One of the outstanding characteristics of OD that distinguishes it from most other improvement programs is that it is based on a "helping relationship." The change agent is not a physician to the organization's ills; he does not examine the "patient," make a *diagnosis*, and write a prescription. Nor does he try to teach organizational members a new inventory of knowledge which they then transfer to the job situation. Using theory and methods drawn from such behavioral sciences as industrial/organizational psychology, *industrial sociology*, *communication*, *cultural anthropology*, *administrative theory*, *organizational behavior*, *economics*, and *political science*, the change agent's main function is to help the organization define and solve its own problems. The basic method used is known as action research. This approach, which is described in detail later, consists of a preliminary diagnosis, collecting data, feedback of the data to the client, data exploration by the client group, action planning based on the data, and taking action.

Systems Context: OD deals with a total system — the organization as a whole, including its relevant environment — or with a subsystem or systems — departments or work groups — in the context of the total system. Parts of systems, for example, individuals, cliques, structures, norms, values, and products are not considered in isolation; the principle of interdependency, that is, that change in one part of a system affects the other parts, is fully recognized. Thus, OD interventions focus on the total culture and cultural processes of organizations. The focus is also on groups, since the relevant behavior of individuals in organizations and groups is generally a product of group influences rather than personality.

Improved Organizational Performance: The objective of OD is to improve the organization's capacity to handle its internal and external functioning and relationships. This would include such things as improved interpersonal and group processes, more effective communication, enhanced ability to cope with organizational problems of all kinds, more effective decision processes, more appropriate leadership style, improved skill in dealing with destructive conflict, and higher levels of trust and cooperation among organizational members. These objectives stem from a value system based on an optimistic view of the nature of man — that man in a supportive environment is capable of achieving higher levels of development and accomplishment. Also essential to organization development and effectiveness is the scientific method — inquiry, a rigorous search for causes, experimental testing of hypotheses, and review of results. Finally, the democratic process is viewed as having a legitimate, and perhaps dominant, role in the highly effective organization.

Organizational Self-Renewal: The ultimate aim of the outside OD practitioner is to "work himself out of a job" by leaving the client organization with a set of tools, behaviors, attitudes, and an action plan with which to monitor its own state of health and to take corrective steps toward its own renewal and development. This is consistent with the systems concept of feedback as a regulatory and corrective mechanism.

The term "Organization Development" is often used interchangeably with *Organizational effectiveness*, especially when used as the name of a department or a part of the *Human Resources* function within an organization. Organization Development is a growing field that is responsive to many new approaches including *Positive Adult Development*.

Early development

Kurt Lewin played a key role in the evolution of organization development as it is known today. As early as *World War II*, Lewin experimented with a collaborative change process (involving himself as consultant and a client group) based on a three-step process of planning, taking action, and measuring results. This was the forerunner of action research, an important element of OD, which will be discussed in detail later in Unit 9. Lewin then participated in the beginnings of laboratory training, or *T-groups*, and, after his death in 1947, his close associates helped to develop survey-research methods at the *University of Michigan*. These procedures becamc important parts of OD as developments in this field continued at the *National Training Laboratories* and in growing numbers of universities and private consulting firms across the country.

The failure of off-site laboratory training to live up to its early promise was one of the important forces stimulating the development of OD. Laboratory training is learning from a person's "here and now" experience as a member of an ongoing training group. Such groups usually meet without a specific agenda. Their purpose is for the members to learn about themselves from their spontaneous "here and now" responses to an ambiguous hypothetical situation. Problems of *leadership*, structure, status, *communication*, and self-serving behavior typically arise in such a group. The members have an opportunity to learn something about themselves and to practice such skills as listening, observing others, and functioning as effective group members.

As formerly practiced (and occasionally still practiced for special purposes), laboratory training was conducted in "stranger groups," or groups composed of individuals from different organizations, situations, and backgrounds. A major difficulty developed, however, in transferring knowledge gained from these "stranger labs" to the actual situation "back home". This required a transfer between two different cultures, the relatively safe and protected environment of the *T-group* (or training group) and the give-and-take of the organizational environment with its traditional values. This led the early pioneers in this type of learning to begin to apply it to "family groups" — that is, groups located within an organization. From this shift in the locale of the training site and the realization that culture was an important factor in influencing group members (along with some other developments in the behavioral sciences) emerged the concept of organization development.

Modern development

In recent years, serious questioning has emerged about the relevance of OD to managing change in modern organizations. The need for "reinventing" the field has become a topic that even some of its "founding fathers" are discussing critically.

With this call for reinvention and change, scholars have begun to examine organizational development from an emotion-based standpoint. For example, deKlerk (2007) writes about how emotional trauma can negatively affect performance. Due to downsizing, outsourcing, mergers, restructuring, continual changes, invasions of privacy, harassment, and abuses of power, many employees experience the emotions of aggression, anxiety, apprehension, cynicism, and fear, which can lead to performance decreases. deKlerk (2007) suggests that in order to heal the trauma and increase performance, O.D. practitioners must acknowledge the existence of the trauma, provide a safe place for employees to discuss their feelings, symbolize the trauma and put it into perspective, and then allow for and deal with the emotional responses. One method of achieving this is by having employees draw pictures of what they feel about the situation, and then having them explain their drawings with each other. Drawing pictures is beneficial because it allows employees to express emotions they normally would not be able to put into words. Also, drawings often prompt active participation in the activity, as everyone is required to draw a picture and then discuss its meaning.

OD interventions

This section describes some of the principal learning processes or interventions in the "action" stage. Interventions are structured activities used individually or in combination by the members of a client *system* to improve their social or task *performance*. They may be introduced by a change agent as part of an improvement program, or they may be used by the client following a program to check on the state of the organization's health, or to effect necessary changes in its own behavior. "Structured activities" mean such diverse procedures as experiential exercises, questionnaires, attitude surveys, interviews, relevant group discussions, and even lunchtime meetings between the change agent and a member of the client *organization*. Every action that influences an organization's improvement program in a change agent-client system relationship can be said to be an intervention.

There are many possible intervention strategies from which to choose. Several assumptions about the nature and functioning of *organizations* are made in the choice of a particular strategy. *Beckhard* lists six such assumptions:

1. The basic building blocks of an *organization* are *groups* (*teams*). Therefore, the basic units of change are groups, not individuals.
2. An always relevant change goal is the reduction of inappropriate *competition* between parts of the organization and the development of a more collaborative condition.
3. Decision making in a healthy organization is located where the information sources are, rather than in a particular role or level of *hierarchy*.
4. Organizations, subunits of organizations, and individuals continuously manage their affairs against goals. Controls are interim measurements, not the basis of managerial strategy.
5. One goal of a healthy organization is to develop generally open *communication*, mutual trust, and *confidence* between and across levels.
6. People support what they help create. People affected by a change must be allowed active participation and a sense of ownership in the planning and conduct of the change.

Interventions range from those designed to improve the *effectiveness* of individuals through those designed to deal with teams and groups, intergroup relations, and the total organization. There are interventions that focus on task issues (what people do), and those that focus on process issues (how people go about doing it). Finally, interventions may be roughly classified according to which change mechanism they tend to emphasize: for example, feedback, awareness of changing cultural norms, interaction and *communication*, *conflict*, and *education* through either new knowledge or skill practice.

One of the most difficult tasks confronting the change agent is to help create in the *client* system a safe climate for learning and change. In a favorable climate, human learning builds on itself and continues indefinitely during man's lifetime. Out of new *behavior*, new dilemmas and problems emerge as the spiral continues upward to new levels. In an unfavorable climate, in contrast, learning is far less certain, and in an atmosphere of psychological threat, it often stops altogether. Unfreezing old ways can be inhibited in *organizations* because the climate makes employees feel that it is inappropriate to reveal true *feelings*, even though such revelations could be constructive. In an inhibited atmosphere, therefore, necessary feedback is not available. Also, trying out new ways may be viewed as risky because it violates established norms. Such an organization may also be constrained because of the law of systems: If one part changes, other parts will become involved. Hence, it is easier to maintain the status quo. Hierarchical authority, *specialization*, span of control, and other characteristics of formal systems also discourage experimentation.

The change agent must address himself to all of these hazards and obstacles. Some of the things which will help him are:

1. A real need in the *client* system to change
2. Genuine support from management
3. Setting a personal example: listening, supporting behavior
4. A sound background in the behavioral sciences

5. A working knowledge of systems theory
6. A belief in man as a rational, self-educating being fully capable of learning better ways to do things.

HRD Committee

Committees are ubiquitous. They exist in all kinds of organizations and serve many different purposes. A committee is a group of persons, either elected or appointed, created to perform some function or mission. A group of people called together for one meeting does not constitute a committee. A committee has an existence of its own, a chairman, designated members, a defined purpose, and often an agreed upon set of operating procedures.

HRD Committees tap the expertise of people from varied backgrounds. In addition to problem-solving, the committees can also provide valuable training and self-development to its members. The members acquire specific knowledge about organizational matters, they gain perspective and understanding, and may improve their skills at the give and take of group interaction.

The HRD Committee is a Specialized Committee function in accordance with the aims and objectives of the International Cooperative Alliance and the policies and decisions of the ICA General Assembly.

In the ICA Policy on Human Resource Development in Co-operatives (adopted in 1990), the concept of HRD in co-operatives is defined as follows:

"The concept of HRD in co-operatives means all the planned information, education, training, mobilisation and manpower development activities undertaken by co-operatives so as to create economically efficient organizations capable of providing services required by their members."

Aims and Objectives of HRD Committee

- To promote and support the initiation and furtherance of HRD programmes within cooperatives and co-operative organizations at global, regional, national and local levels, so as to enhance their social and economic effectiveness.

Functions

The functions of the HRD Committee shall be:

A. to promote the systematic dissemination of information on the significance of HRD for co-operatives and co-operative organizations and to promote HRD activities wherever relevant;

B. to help further the development of appropriate HRD frameworks within each of the regions of the ICA and to assist national projects and programmes in the sphere of HRD, in collaboration and agreement with regional HRD committees;

C. to ensure the inclusion of HRD related activities as an integral element on the agendas of ICA Regional and General Assemblies;

D. to facilitate effective interaction among the ICA regional HRD frameworks, including the organization of joint conferences;

E. to establish effective network relationships among all relevant bodies within and outside of ICA engaged in co-operative HRD;

F. to facilitate through such network relationships the exchange of experience, educational and training material, staff, management and personnel, information and other relevant elements among institutions and bodies concerned with cooperative HRD;

G. to initiate contact and interaction with relevant non-ICA frameworks concerned with co-operative HRD including those drawn from the academic world, from the world of international organizations and civil society, communities, etc.;

H. to facilitate periodic reviews of HRD systems utilized by co-operative movements worldwide; to help identify areas of best HRD practice as well as needs for assistance in this regard; to help develop HRD programmes which further the realization of co-operative values and principles in co-operative enterprise as well as those which enhance managerial efficiency and the ability to achieve business objectives in co-operatives; to help promote strategies and approaches furthering a greater degree of member participation in co-operative management and organization and in general to identify areas appropriate for HRD training, research and technical assistance at global level;

I. to develop effective working relationships with other ICA specialized bodies, Particularly with the committees concerned with research and with communication;

J. to carry out any other activities relevant and/or conducive to the promotion and furtherance of the aims and objectives of the HRD Committee.

Membership

a. The members of the HRD Committee should be persons responsible for and actively involved in co-operative HRD activities;

b. The HRD Committee may decide to invite members actively involved in co-operative HRD to become institutional members;

c. In general, observers both from ICA members and non-member organizations may be invited to participate in HRD Committee meetings and/or activities;

d. International organizations engaged, on an ongoing basis, in co-operative HRD related activities such as ILO, FAO, UNESCO, COPAC, etc., could be asked to send observers to relevant HRD Committee meetings and activities;

e. The Director-General of ICA and the Directors of the ICA Regional Offices, or nominees designated by the Director-General and/or the Directors of the ICA Regional Offices, could be invited to attend meetings of the HRD Committee;

f. Chairpersons and Secretaries of other regional HRD committees could be invited to attend meetings of the HRD Committee;

g. Members could serve on the HRD Committee from one General Assembly meeting to the next and may be renominated for further terms;

h. The secretariat shall keep a register of members;

i. Participation in activities may carry a fee to be determined from time to time.

For Example: The office of the Global HRD Committee is at the ICA head office in Geneva.

Officers

a. The Global HRD Committee elects an Executive Committee consisting of a Chairperson, four Vice Chairpersons who will be the Chairpersons of the regional HRD committees, a Secretary and five Committee members. Every possible effort should be made to ensure that the Executive Committee include members from the widest possible geographic scope, and women are included in significant proportion among their numbers.

b. Executive Committee members serve for a period of four years. Elections are held at every second General Assembly meeting. Retiring officers shall be eligible for reelection.

Meetings

a. The Global HRD Committee meets regularly once every two years at the time and place of each meeting of the ICA General Assembly and at other times and places when necessary.

b. The Executive Committee of the Global HRD Committee meets once each year, at the time and place of the meetings of the General Assembly and at the time and place of one of the Regional Assemblies in the years when there is no General Assembly meeting. It may also meet at other times and places if and when necessary.

c. Meetings of the Global HRD Committee will be convened by the Executive Committee. The Secretary of the Global HRD Committee informs its members in good time of the date, place and agenda of the meetings and provides them with relevant reports, background material, etc. Meetings of the Executive Committee is convened by the Chairperson, Vice Chairpersons and Secretary.

d. The language of the meetings of the Global HRD Committee and its Executive Committee is English. Participants requiring interpretation in any other language may be accompanied by personal interpreters at their own expense.

e. The Global HRD Committee and its Executive Committee will have their own rules of procedure and conduct. They are be guided by the rules and procedures of the ICA.

f. The quorum of the Global HRD Committee has to consist of members from seven countries. The quorum for a meeting of the Executive committee has to consist of four members. In the absence of the Chairperson, one of the Vice Chairpersons shall chair the meetings of the Global HRD Committee and/or of the Executive Committee. In the absence of both the Chairperson and the Vice Chairpersons, members of the Global HRD Committee and/or Executive Committee shall elect a member to serve as chairperson for the meeting.

Reporting

a. The Global HRD Committee has to report to each session of the General Assembly as to its activities, programmes, etc.

b. Written reports have to be submitted to appropriate ICA bodies as requested and/or required.

c. The Executive Committee reports, verbally and in writing, to each of the meetings of the Global HRD Committee on its activities, and in between meetings on matters of importance using various means of communication.

Financing

a. Participation in meetings and activities of the Global HRD Committee and its Executive is on a self-financing basis.

b. The financial year of the Global HRD Committee is the calendar year.

c. The Executive Committee has to present appropriate financial reports to the Global HRD Committee.

d. The accounts of the Global HRD Committee is audited annually in accordance with ICA standards.

e. As an ICA Specialized Committee, the Global HRD Committee seeks appropriate institutional support from ICA when relevant.

To give a drive and thrust for an effort in organizational development, it was found necessary to have a committee with top management support. A Human Resource Committee (HRC) is constituted with the main objective of bringing about an integrated development of employees.

HRD FOR WOMEN AN OPINION STUDY

The status of **women in India** has been subject to many great changes over the past few millennia. From a largely unknown status in ancient times through the low points of the medieval period, to the promotion of *equal rights* by many reformers, the history of women in *India* has been eventful:

Workforce participation

Contrary to the common perception, a large percent of women in India work. The National data collection agencies accept the fact that there is a serious under-estimation of women's contribution as workers. However, there are far fewer women in the paid workforce than there are men. In urban India Women have impressive number in the workforce. As an example at software industry 30% of the workforce is female. They are at par with their male counter parts in terms of wages, position at the work place.

In rural India, agriculture and allied industrial sectors employ as much as 89.5% of the total female labour. In overall farm production, women's average contribution is estimated at 55% to 66% of the total labour. According to a 1991 World Bank report, women accounted for 94% of total employment in dairy production in India. Women constitute 51% of the total employed in forest-based small-scale enterprises.

One of the most famous female business success stories is the *Shri Mahila Griha Udyog Lijjat Papad*. In 2006, *Kiran Mazumdar-Shaw*, who started Biocon - one of India's first biotech companies, was rated India's richest woman. Lalita Gupte and Kalpana Morparia (both were the only businesswomen in India who made the list of the Forbes World's Most Powerful Women), run India's second-largest bank, *ICICI Bank*.

There is no doubt that we are in the midst of a great revolution in the history of women. The evidence is everywhere; the voice of women is increasingly heard in Parliament, courts and in the streets.

While women in the West had to fight for over a century to get some of their basic rights, like the right to vote, the Constitution of India gave women equal rights with men from the beginning. Unfortunately, women in this country are mostly unaware of their rights because of illiteracy and the oppressive tradition. Names like Kalpana Chawla: The Indian born, who fought her way up into NASA and was the first women in space, and Indira Gandhi: The Iron Woman of India was the Prime Minister of the Nation, Beauty Queens like Aishwarya Rai and Susmita Sen, and Mother Teresa are not representative of the condition of Indian women. According to last census held in 2001, the percentage of female literacy in the country is 54.16%. The literacy rate in the country has increased from 18.33% in 1951 to 65.38% as per 2001 census. The female literacy rate has also increased from 8.86% in 1951 to 54.16%. It is noticed that the female literacy rate during the period 1991-2001 increased by 14.87% whereas male literacy rate rose by 11.72%. Hence the female literacy rate actually increased by 3.15% more compared to male literacy rate.

Factors Responsible for Poor Female Literacy Rate

Historically, a variety of factors have been found to be responsible for poor female literate rate, viz

- Gender based inequality.
- Social discrimination and economic exploitation.
- Occupation of girl child in domestic chores.
- Low enrolment of girls in schools.
- Low retention rate and high dropout rate.

Strategies adopted by the HRD, Government of India, for increasing **Women Empowerment** in the Country:

The main strategies adopted by the HRD, Government of India, for women empowerment in the country include:

1. National Literacy Mission for imparting functional literacy
2. Universalisation for Elementary Education
3. Non-Formal Education

HRD and Women

The provision of educational opportunities for women has been an important part of the national endeavor in the field of education since India's Independence. Though these endeavors did yield significant results, gender disparity persists with uncompromising tenacity, more so in the rural areas and among the disadvantaged communities. This is not only a matter of national anxiety and concern but also a matter of national conscience. It is with this concern that the Government of India launched the National Literacy Mission in 1988 for eradication of adult illiteracy. Since women account for an overwhelming percentage of the total number of illiterates, the National Literacy Mission is for all practical purposes a Mission of imparting functional literacy to women. Total literacy campaigns launched since 1988 under the aegis of the National emphasis on making efforts to:

- Create an environment where women demand knowledge and information, empowering themselves to change their lives.
- Inculcate in women the confidence that change is possible, if women work collectively.
- Spread the message that education of women is a pre-condition for fighting against their oppression.
- Highlight the plight of the girl child and stress the need for Universalisation of elementary education as a way of addressing the issue.

Some of the significant ways in which the HRD can contribute to the promotion of women's empowerment and they are as follows:

Heightened Social Awareness

HRD programs has heightened social awareness among women regarding the importance of education, both for themselves as well as for their children. Large numbers of women have been participating whole-heartedly in the literacy campaigns as learners and volunteers. Because of the campaign mode and creation of a positive environment for literacy, women receive a social sanction to participate in the literacy programs. As women came out of their homes and take part in the campaigns with great enthusiasm, they acquire a heightened sense of self-awareness and desire to gain knowledge of host of women's issues.

Increased School Enrolment

The HRD programs have also motivated and encouraged women learners to educate their children, particularly girls by enrolling them in formal schools. An evaluation study of the literacy campaign ion Birbhum District shows that the biggest achievement of the adult literacy program in Birbhum has been its impact on girls' education. The confidence of the girls, as they perform drill or play football, is the result of the awareness among neo-literate parents that girls need to be educated and outgoing. The need to provide equal opportunity to both girls and boys has also had effect of generating greater demand for the quantity to both girls and boys has also had effect of generating greater demand for the quantity and quality of primary schooling.

Increase in Self-Confidence and Personality Development

The literacy classes conducted under HRD programs have given women as opportunity to break the isolation which is socially structured into their lives, giving them a chance to meet other women and learn collectively- rather than learn singly as individuals. The newly acquired literacy skills have enhanced their ability to solve family problems and learn new skills. Women are communicating how they have started feeling more confident, how their articulation has improved, how they have become more discerning and how they have learnt to function autonomously.

Gender Equity and Women's Empowerment

HRD programs have provided illiterate adult women, who have been denied access to formal schooling, with a great opportunity for reading, writing, increasing awareness levels and skills training. Literacy campaigns have thus actively promoted gender equity and have sought to empower them as to decision making about themselves, their families and their communities. The impact of literacy on women's life has often been dramatic. Experiences of Poddukuttai in Tamil Nadu (where women learnt how to bicycle and acquired ownership right in stone quarries) and Nellore in Andhra Pradesh (where a lesson in the literacy Primer inspired women to launch anti-arrack agitation that later engulfed the entire district and the state) have shown how women have been empowered at individual and collective levels as a result of their participation.

States in the Family

HRD programs have played a significant role in improving the status of women within their won families. Whereas traditionally, women have little say in the family decision making, they, through participation in literacy programs, have begun to express their newly found self-belief in having say both within and without the family.

Educational Equality

Another area in which women's equality has shown a major improvement as a result of adult literacy programs is the area of enrolment of boys and girls in schools. As a result of higher participation of women in literacy campaigns, the gender gap in literacy levels is gradually getting reduced. Even more significant is the fact that disparity in enrolment of boys and girls in neo-literate households is much lowered compared to the non-literate householders.

Women as Entrepreneurs

Participation of women in HRD programs has opened several opportunities for neo-literate women to step out of the households and involve themselves in some enterprise or a new vocation. The Dumka campaign in Bihar has demonstrated how literacy campaign has helped women has demonstrated how literacy campaign has helped women to take charge of their lives. They have formed a group called "Joga Behna" (Awake sister), which tries to sensitize the women to the need of collective action against social ills. These women have also set up "Didi Bank" (Sister Bank) which promotes the habits of thrifts and savings. Here women have also learnt to maintain hand pump thereby breaking their dependence for repair on mechanics from outside the village.

Household Savings and Access to Credit

In almost all the districts, the HRD programs have gone beyond the transaction of mere literacy skills and have served to enhance knowledge and skills for better management of expenditure and improving earning capacities. In several districts, the women participants in literacy campaigns have begun to set aside their earnings not only in regular banks but also in specially thrift societies. Such societies, as for example in Dumka are run by the women themselves.

Health and Hygiene

HRD programs in most districts have taken up health and hygiene issues as an integral component of adult education programs. Literacy campaigns have helped to spread knowledge about health care and nutrition, thereby enabling mothers to keep their family in better health and to care better for their children. Literacy campaigns have also disseminated information for creating awareness about problems of early marriage, spacing and small family norms.

Small Scale Sector

The **small-scale** industries **sector** plays a vital role in the growth of the country. The exports from SSI **sector** have been clocking excellent growth rates in the country. The opportunities in the **small scale sector** are enormous. The phenomenal growth of industries in the **Small Scale sector** has been striking. Government Policies, schemes and export promotion programs for **Small Scale Sector** in India, Export-Import Policy for **Small Scale Sector**, The phenomenal growth of industries in the Small Scale sector has been striking feature in the economic development of the country since independence. It has contributed to the overall growth or the Gross Domestic Product as well as in terms of employment generation and export.

One of the measure of the policy support for promoting small scale industries is the policy of reservation of economically viable and technically feasible items for exclusive manufacture in the small scale sector. The policy of reservation initiated in 1967 primarily as promotional and protective measure vis-a-vis the large scale sector, grants protection to small scale sector, the only exception being the case of large units which undertake minimum level of exports as 75 per cent of their total production. The IDR Act was amended in March, 1984 empowering Government to reserve items for the small scale sector. Reservation/De-reservation of items for manufacture in the small scale sector is a continuing process regularly monitored by an Advisory committee on Reservation constituted under the IDR Act. at present the total number of items reserved for small scale sector are 799 as on 29.06.2001

The small scale sector has acquired a prominent place in the socio-economic development of the country during the past six decades. It has contributed to the overall growth of the gross domestic product as well as in terms of employment generation and export. Performance of the small scale sector, which forms a part of total industrial sector, therefore, has direct impact on the growth of the national economy.

There has been a steady increase in the number of SSI units, their production, employment and exports over the years, from 19,58,000 units in 1990-91, the number of units has increased to 33, 70,000 units in the year 2000-01. On the production front also, there has been a steady increase over the previous years ranging between 7%-10% during the period 1990-91 to 1994-95. The increase was 11.4% and 11.3% in 1995-96 and 1996-97 respectively. In 1997-98 the increase over the previous year was registered at 8.43%. The increase in the year 1998-99 & 1999-2000 were 7.7%, and 8.16% respectively. The estimated increase for -2000-01 is 8.09%.

On the exports front there has been an increase with Rs. 9,664 crores worth exports in 1990-91 which has over the years increased to Rs. 43,946 crores in 1997-98. The figures of exports for the years 1998-99 and 1999-00 are Rs. 48, 979 crores and Rs. 54,200.47 crores respectively, with the increase over the previous years in percentage terms being 11.45% and 10.66% respectively. The provisional/estimated figure for export for the year 2000-01 is 59,978 crore showing an increase of 10.66% over 1999-2000.

Hon'ble Prime Minister announced a Comprehensive Policy Package for SSI sector on 30th August 2000 at Vigyan Bhawan, New Delhi. The package included among other things Government of India's resolve to go in for a fresh census covering, inter-alia the incidence of sickness and its causes. Immediately after the announcement a Steering Committee has been constituted under the Chairmanship of Secretary (SSI & ARI) to look into all the aspects relating to the conduct of census by the Office of the Development Commissioner (SSI).

HRD and Small scale sector

Prime Minister's Rozgar Yojana was launched on 2nd Oct. 1993. The Scheme envisages to create one million employment opportunities by assisting for setting up of nearly 7 lakh tiny micro enterprises during the remaining period of the Eighth Five Year Plan. The Scheme is continuing in 9th Plan. The Scheme aimed at assisting the eligible youth in setting up self-employment ventures in industry, service and business sectors.

Over the last five decades, the small scale industries (SSI) sector has acquired a place of prominence in the economy of the country. It has contributed significantly to the growth of the Gross Domestic Product (GDP), employment generation and exports. The sector now includes not only SSI units but also small scale service and business enterprises (SSSBEs) and is thus referred to as the small enterprises sector. During 2000-01 to 2004-05, the SSI sector registered continuous growth in the number of units, production, employment and even exports (till 2002-03). During this period, the average annual growth in the number of units was around 4.1 per cent, while employment grew by 4.4 per cent annually. Further, the average annual growth in production, at current and constant prices, was 10.6 per cent and 7.6 per cent respectively. The small enterprises sector, however, faces several problems, which hamper it in achieving its full growth potential. Some of the major problems faced by the sector are access to timely and adequate credit, technological obsolescence, infrastructural bottlenecks, marketing constraints and a plethora of rules and regulations. Some policy initiatives taken during the year may help promote and develop the SSI sector The National Commission on Enterprises in the Unorganized/Informal Sector was set up in September 2004. The Commission will, inter-alia, recommend measures considered necessary for improvement in the productivity of these enterprises, generation of large scale employment opportunities on a sustainable basis, linkage of the sector to institutional framework in areas like credit, raw material supply, infrastructure, technology upgradation, marketing facilities and skill development 85 items reserved for exclusive manufacture in the SSI sector were dereserved in October 2004. The total number of reserved items now stands at 605.

A new "Promotional Package for small enterprises" is being formulated. This would include measures to provide adequate credit, incentives for technology upgradation, infrastructural and marketing facilities, etc.

Family-owned small businesses constitute a large proportion of the overall small business population of industrially developed and developing countries. A great deal of theoretical and practical knowledge exists on various aspects of small business growth and development, including: management, marketing, finance, production, research and development. There exists, however, a paucity of comparative research on the training and HRD strategies of small family and non-family businesses. This article sets out to redress this imbalance in current small business research. It outlines the preliminary results of a recent study that focused on the training and HRD needs of a randomly selected sample of 6,000 small businesses in Great Britain. The data shows that there are considerable differences in owner/manager attitudes and approaches towards the training needs of family members employed in a business as compared to non-family employees. The results suggest that these differences could have a significant influence upon the competitive strategies of family and non-family owned small businesses.

The small scale sector has emerged as a dynamic and vibrant sector of the Indian economy. It has contributed significantly to the realisation of the socio-economic objectives of growth in employment and exports, fostering entrepreneurship and ensuring industrial dispersal.

During 1999-2000, the production from SSIs was estimated at Rs. 5,78,470 crores and provided employment to more than 177 lakh persons in the 32 lakh SSI units spread throughout the country. Exports from SSIs have been estimated at Rs. 48,979 crores in 1998-99. The Small Scale Sector has been contributing about 40% of industrial production and 35% of total direct exports. This sector has been maintaining, by and large, a higher growth than the industrial sector as a whole. The share of this sector in employment generation is next only to agriculture.

The ongoing process of liberalisation warrants due attention to be given to the medium and long term interests of the small scale sector. This sector, nurtured hitherto in a protective framework, needs to be enabled to take on the challenges posed to it by the process of liberalisation and globalisation.

The HRD, Government is conscious of the role and importance of Small Scale Industries in strengthening our economic performance and is therefore committed to putting in place a policy framework that would address the problems of this sector and help it become internationally competitive. In recognition of the importance of the SSI sector and to give focused attention Government has created a separate ***Ministry for Small Scale Industries and Agro & Rural Industries*** in October 1999.

The small scale sector plays a vital role in the growth of a country. The opportunities in the small scale sector are enormous due to:

- The phenomenal growth of industries in the Small Scale sector has been striking feature in the economic development of the country since independence. It has contributed to the overall growth or the Gross Domestic Product as well as in terms of employment generation and export.
- The small scale sector has played a very important role in the socio-economic development of the country during the past 50 years. It has significantly contributed to the overall growth in terms of the Gross Domestic Product (GDP), employment generation and exports. The performance of the small scale sector, therefore, has a direct impact on the growth of the overall economy.

HRD AND FUNCTIONAL LITERACY

The traditional definition of **literacy** is considered to be the ability to use *language* to *read*, *write*, *listen*, and *speak*. In modern contexts, the word refers to reading and writing at a level adequate for *communication*, or at a level that lets one understand and communicate ideas in a literate *society*, so as to take part in that society.

The *United Nations Educational, Scientific and Cultural Organization (UNESCO)* has drafted the following definition: "'Literacy' is the ability to identify, understand, interpret, create, communicate, compute and use printed and written materials associated with varying contexts. Literacy involves a continuum of learning to enable an individual to achieve his or her goals, to develop his or her knowledge and potential, and to participate fully in the wider society." In modern times, illiteracy is seen as a social problem to be solved through education.

Traditional definitions of literacy consider the ability to "read, write, spell, listen, and speak." Since the 1980s, some have argued that literacy is ideological, which means that literacy always exists in a context, in tandem with the values associated with that context. Prior work viewed literacy as existing autonomously.

Some have argued that the definition of literacy should be expanded. For example, in the United States, the *National Council of Teachers of English* and the *International Reading Association* have added "visually representing" to the traditional list of competencies. Similarly, in Scotland, literacy has been defined as: "The ability to read and write and use numeracy, to handle information, to express ideas and opinions, to make decisions and solve problems, as family members, workers, citizens and lifelong learners."

A basic literacy standard in many societies is the ability to read the newspaper. Increasingly, communication in commerce or society in general requires the ability to use computers and other digital technologies. Since the 1990s, when the *Internet* came into wide use in the United States, some have asserted that the definition of literacy should include the ability to use tools such as *web browsers*, *word processing* programs, and *text messages*. Similar expanded skill sets have been called *multimedia literacy*, *computer literacy*, *information literacy*, and *technacy*.

Taking account of the fact that a large part of the benefits of literacy obtain from having access to a literate person in the household, a recent literature in economics, starting with the work of Kaushik

Basu and James Foster, distinguishes between a 'proximate illiterate' and an 'isolated illiterate'. The former refers to an illiterate person who lives in a household with other literates and the latter to an illiterate who lives in a household of all illiterates. What is of concern is that lots of people in poor nations are not just illiterates but isolated illiterates.

Traditionally literacy has been commonly defined as the ability to read and write at an adequate level of proficiency that is necessary for communication. More recently however, literacy has taken on several meanings. Technological literacy, mathematical literacy, and visual literacy are just a few examples. While it may be difficult to gauge the degree to which literacy has an impact on an individual's overall happiness, one can easily infer that an increase in literacy will lead to the improvement of an individual's life and the development of societies.

Functional literacy

The concept of "**functional literacy**" has emerged to describe the use of basic skills in specific contexts. The concept of functional literacy is controversial, however. Because functional literacy is determined by external standards and criteria, it removes the literacy judgment from the individual's cultural group and social setting. Critics feel such external criteria tend to reflect the bias of their developers rather than the values and norms of the individual's social and cultural group.

Literacy is not merely about basic skills of reading and writing; it is about providing individuals with the capabilities for understanding their lives and social environment as well as equipping them with problem-solving skills. Literacy, therefore, is a foundation of human resources development and is critical to alleviating poverty and to enhancing the general quality of life of the people. Traditionally literacy has been commonly defined as the ability to read and write at an adequate level of proficiency that is necessary for communication. More recently however, literacy has taken on several meanings. Technological literacy, mathematical literacy, and visual literacy are just a few examples. While it may be difficult to gauge the degree to which literacy has an impact on an individual's overall happiness, one can easily infer that an increase in literacy will lead to the improvement of an individual's life and the development of societies.

While in developed nations, the majority of the population over the age of 17 possesses basic literacy skills in reading and writing,, the rate of literacy in developing nations is much lower. This lack of widespread literacy hinders the further development of such nations. International agencies like UNESCO are campaigning to raise literacy rates worldwide. While progress has been made and literacy rates have increased, the growth in population worldwide has led to a further expansion of illiterate individuals. UNESCO has found a correlation between illiteracy and poverty, low life expectancy, and political oppression.

Literacy campaigns around the world also include programs to increase the level of adult literacy. Increasing literacy rates among adults can serve several purposes. Equipping adults with basic literacy skills can enable them to be more proactive when it comes to their child's education. As this works to increase literacy, political conditions in oppressive countries may improve. Moreover an increase in literate adults means an increase in individuals campaigning for education as a fundamental human right.

Sri Lanka is an example of a developing nation that has shown a dramatic increase in literacy. Sri Lanka has a literacy rate of 96%, one of the highest literacy rates in all of South Asia and much higher than that expected of a developing country. This can be attributed to the country's policy of providing free education to all children regardless of income. Additionally, the illiteracy rate for adults 15-24 is only 4.4% according to the 2001 census. (*wiki*)

Functional illiteracy

Functional illiteracy is a term used to describe reading and *writing* skills that are inadequate to cope with the demands of everyday life. This is contrasted with illiteracy in the strict sense, meaning the inability to read or write simple sentences in any language.

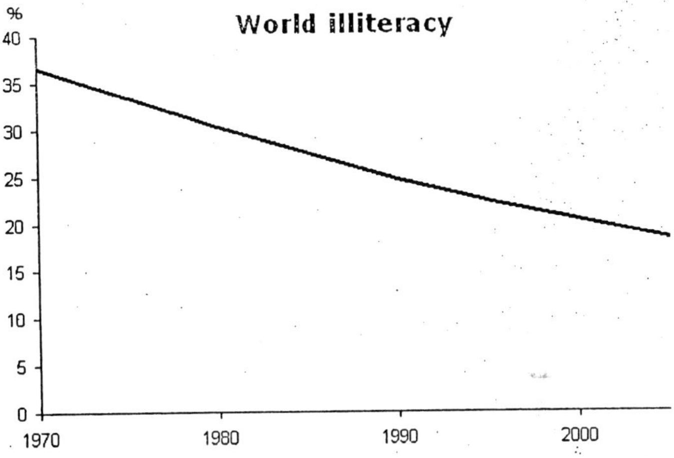

World illiteracy halved between 1970 and 2005

80% of the world population was literate in 1998 by the United Nations definition - the ability to read and write a simple sentence in a language. Using a definition of: "age 15 and over can read and write", the U.S. *CIA World Factbook* estimated in 2007 that the overall world literacy rate was 82%.

Literacy rates can vary widely from country to country or region to region. This often coincides with the region's *wealth* or *urbanization*, though many factors play a role, such as social customs which limit the education of females in some countries.

Many policy analysts consider literacy rates a crucial measure of a region's *human capital*. This claim is made on the grounds that literate people can be trained less expensively than illiterate people, generally have a higher socio-economic status and enjoy better health and employment prospects. Policy makers also argue that literacy increases job opportunities and access to *higher education*. In *Kerala, India*, for example, female and child mortality rates declined dramatically in the 1960s, when girls who were schooled according to the *education reforms* after 1948 began to raise families. Recent researchers argue, however, that such correlations may have more to do with the overall effects of schooling rather than literacy alone. In addition to the potential for literacy to increase wealth, wealth may promote literacy, through cultural norms and easier access to schools and tutoring services.

Characteristics

An *illiterate* person cannot read or write at all, for all practical purposes. A *functionally illiterate* person can read and possibly write simple sentences with a limited vocabulary, but cannot read or write well enough to deal with the everyday requirements of life in his own society.

For example, an illiterate person may not even understand the written words *cat* or *dog,* and may not even recognize the letters of the alphabet. A functionally illiterate person may well understand these words and more, but cannot read well enough to understand the things he must read in order to get by in his daily life, such as job advertisements, past-due notices, newspaper articles, complex signs and posters, etc.

While pure illiteracy has approximately the same characteristics worldwide, the characteristics of functional illiteracy vary from one culture to another, as some cultures require better reading and writing skills than others. A reading level that might be sufficient to make a farmer functionally literate in a rural area of a developing country might qualify as functional illiteracy in an urban area of a technologically advanced country.

Those who are functionally illiterate may be subject to social intimidation, health risks, stress, low income, and other pitfalls associated with their reading and writing deficits. Their inability to function normally in society because of their functional illiteracy may increase the friction they experience with the mainstream of society, and thereby increase the likelihood that they will become involved in antisocial activities such as crime, or self-destructive activities.

In the United States, according to *Business* magazine, an estimated 15 million functionally illiterate adults held jobs at the beginning of the 21st century. The *American Council of Life Insurers* reported that 75% of the *Fortune 500* companies provide some level of remedial training for their workers. All over the U.S.A. 30 million (14% of adults) are unable to perform simple and everyday literacy activities.

A Literacy at Work study, published by the Northeast Institute, in 2001, found that business losses attributed to basic skill deficiencies run into billions of dollars a year due to low productivity, errors, and accidents attributed to functional illiteracy.

Functional illiteracy is a serious problem for Human Resource Development. Literacy is an instrument for development. It has both direct and indirect benefits.

It helps an individual in the following ways:

- It equips the individual with capabilities to transact with the changing world, opportunities and problems.
- It helps an individual in having access to information about various aspects relating to one's needs irrespective of the field to which one's needs belong.
- It helps an individual to acquire more knowledge that can make one eligible for high level opportunities which in turn improves the standard of living.
- It helps a person in making decisions that are beneficial to him/ her. These decisions may again relate to the health conditions, economic activities, pursuing leisure and other activities.
- In terms of human resource development literacy installs a new confidence in the individual due to his capabilities to transact with the environment.
- It contributes by helping the individual to participate better in choosing political leaders and in the community activities that may indirectly/ directly affect him.
- Makes one aware of his rights and the means of getting what is due to him.
- Helps a person to make use of the various development and other opportunities offered by his environment.

According to American Management Association (AMA) survey, the areas in which remedial training required for employees are mathematics, reading and writing.

Increase in literacy was found to contribute to increase in investment and in output per worker.

HRD and Functional Literacy

Because HRD programs are developed in response to differing perspectives, they have differing purposes. Two common models are (1) personal development and (2) empowerment and social change.

The personal development model, which predominates in this country, emphasizes individual development. In this model, literacy is viewed as a skill that will enable the adult to change. The role of the educator in the personal development model is that of instructor and counselor.

The empowerment (increasing group or individual ability to control their own lives) and social change model emphasizes making illiterate adults critically aware of social and political realities so that they can make changes in the existing system. In this model, the educator plays the role of facilitator and change agent. While not common in this country, the social change model has been used widely abroad.

The delivery systems for adult literacy programs in this country generally correspond to either the personal development or the social change model.

Such organizations frequently work successfully with those persons who do not participate in more traditional programs serving individuals. The programs are characterized by a collaborative process in which mutually agreeable goals are worked out between the instructor and the students. Frequently, this process is more important than the end product.

Adult illiteracy is a growing problem despite efforts to curb it. Each year, an estimated 2.3 million persons join the pool of those 23 million adults considered to be functionally illiterate. This number includes high school dropouts and "push-outs," legal and illegal immigrants, and refugees (United States Department of Education). The cost of illiteracy in increased participation in welfare programs and unemployment compensation is estimated to be $6 billion a year (Wellborn 1982).

Adult illiteracy is a growing problem despite efforts to curb it. Each year, an estimated 2.3 million persons join the pool of those 23 million adults considered to be functionally illiterate. This number includes high school dropouts and "push-outs," legal and illegal immigrants, and refugees (United States Department of Education). The cost of illiteracy in increased participation in welfare programs and unemployment compensation is estimated to be $6 billion a year (Wellborn 1982). **Human resources** is a term with which organizations describe the combination of traditionally administrative personnel functions with performance, Employee Relations and *resource* planning. The field draws upon concepts developed in Industrial/Organizational Psychology. Human resources has at least two related interpretations depending on context. The original usage derives from *political economy* and *economics*, where it was traditionally called *labor*, one of four *factors of production*. The more common usage within *corporations* and *businesses* refers to the individuals within the firm, and to the portion of the firm's organization that deals with hiring, firing, training, and other personnel issues. This article addresses both definitions.

The objective of HRD is to maximize the return on investment from the organization's human capital and minimize financial risk. It is the responsibility of HRD programs to conduct these activities in an effective, legal, fair, and consistent manner.

SUMMARY

Organization Development is the attempt to influence the members of an organization to expand their candidness with each other about their views of the organization and their experience in it, and to take greater responsibility for their own actions as organization members. The assumption behind OD is that when people pursue both of these objectives simultaneously, they are likely to discover new ways of working together that they experience as more effective for achieving their own and their shared (organizational) goals. And that when this does not happen, such activity helps them to understand why and to make meaningful choices about what to do in light of this understanding. Aims and Objectives of HRD Committee is to promote and support the initiation and furtherance of HRD programmes within cooperatives and co-operative organizations at global, regional, national and local levels, so as to enhance their social and economic effectiveness.

UNIT 6

MODELS IN HUMAN RESOURCE DEVELOPMENT

INTRODUCTION

The first HRD department in the Indian corporate sector was started in 1975 in Larsen & Toubro (L&T), after recommendations by two consultants Udai Pareek and T.V. Rao from Indian Institute of Management. By the mid eighties, the importance of HRD had grown to such an extent, that almost every second organization in India had established an HRD. By the nineties almost every organization had an HR department with the function being fully institutionalized. This has opened up the doors for career development in HRD.

A new professional body called the National HRD Network took birth in 1985, and is comparable to the Organizational Development network in the USA. This body has even established a national level research institution called the Academy of HRD which concentrates on research in various areas of HRD lime models of HRD, HRD systems, barriers to HRD requirement of HRD to deal with social change and so on.

This unit discusses the behavioral model of HRD, career development in HRD, integrated HRD systems, HR and management, barriers to HRD, career path planning, HRD – as the need of the hour and for social change and also research in HRD.

VARIOUS MODELS OF HRD

As HRD came to prominence many models came into existence. Some of these are presented below:

The strategic HR framework: It was formulated by Ulrich and Lake (1990) aims to leverage and/or align HR practices to build critical organizational capabilities that enable an organization to achieve its goals. This approach offers specific tools and paths to identify how a firm can leverage its HR practices. Business strategy, organizational capabilities and HR practices are the three important elements in this model. Dave Ulrich (1997) presented a framework for HR professionals in terms of four key roles: (1) management of strategic human resource (2) management of firm infrastructure (3) management of the employee contribution (4) management of transformation and change.

The activities for management of Firm infrastructure: This includes constant examination to improve the HR practices, HR professionals to act as administrative experts ferative unnecessary cause, improving efficiency and constantly finding new ways to do things better, being effective as administrative experts. They also need to undertake activities leading to continual re-engineering of the work processes they administer. It requires HR professional's desire to deliver efficient HR practices for staffing, training, appraising, and rewarding and otherwise managing the flow of employees includes reasoning, responding and finding ways to provide employees with resources that meet their changing demands. The activities for managing transformation and change include identifying and framing problems, building relationships of trust, solving problems, creating and fulfilling action plans.

The Integrative framework: this framework offered by Yeung and Berman (1997) identifies three paths through which Hr practices can contribute to business performance.: (1) organizational capabilities (2) by improving employee satisfaction and (3) by shaping customer and shareholder satisfaction. Yeung and Berman (1997) argued for dynamic change sin HR measures to refocus on priorities and resources of the HR function. They argued that HR measures should be business measures should be business driven rather than HR driven: impact driven rather than activity driven: forward looking and innovative rather than backward looking: and instead of focusing on individual HR practice the measure should focus on the entire HR system taking into account synergies existing among all HR practices.

Human Capital Appraisal Approach: this approach outlined by Fredmann et al., is based on the belief that there are five stages in the management of human capital: clarification stage, assessment stage, design stage, implementation stage and monitoring stage. They are five areas of human capital management: recruitment, retention and retirement: rewards and performance management: career development, succession planning and training: organizational structure, and human capital enablers. A 5 x 5 matrix using these 5 stages and 5 areas could be used to evaluate and mange the human capital well. For example, in the clarification stage the managers examine the human capital programs to dit into their strategy and overall culture. They may also examine each of the areas to fit into the strategy, etc.

HRD Score Card Approach : A recent approach formulated by Rao (1999) envisages that Hr interventions in order to make the right business impact should be mature in terms of HRD systems, competencies, culture (including styles) and business linkages. The maturity level and the appropriateness of each of the subsystems of HR, the appropriateness of the HR structure and the level of competencies of HR staff line managers, top management, etc., the HRD culture (define in terms of openness, elaboration, trust, autonomy, proaction, authenticity, confrontation and experimentation) and the congruence of the top management, HR staff styles with HRD culture, and the Extent to which all the systems and practices result in employee satisfaction and customer satisfaction, etc., are assessed through a well formulated HRD audit.

P-CMM Approach: Curtis and team (Curtis et al., 1995) developed this approach for soft ware organizations. The People Capability Maturity Model (P-CMM) aims at providing guidance on how to improve the ability of software organizations to attract, develop, motivate, organize, and retain the talent needed to steadily improve their software development capability. The strategic objectives of P-CMM are:

- Improving the capability of software organizations by increasing the capability of the work force.

- Ensuring that the software development capability is an attribute of an organization rather than that of a few individuals.
- Aligning the motivation of individuals with that of the organizations.
- Retaining human assets, i.e., people with critical knowledge and skills within the organization.

BEHAVIORAL MODEL IN HRD

This is built on the foundation of the work of B.F. Skinner, which takes the advantage of human being's ability to modify behavior in response to tasks and feedback. The model is used for a wide variety of applications in HRD, from training, teaching concepts and skills to increasing comfort and relaxation, decreasing phobias, changing habits, and learning to control one's behavior.

Human behavior is the collection of *behaviors* exhibited by *human beings* and influenced by *culture*, *attitudes*, *emotions*, *values*, *ethics*, *authority*, *rapport*, *hypnosis*, *persuasion*, *coercion* and/or *genetics*.

The behavior of *people* (and other *organisms* or even mechanisms) falls within a *range* with some behavior being common, some unusual, some acceptable, and some *outside acceptable limits*. In *sociology*, behavior is considered as having no meaning, being not directed at other people and thus is the most basic human *action*. Behavior should not be mistaken with *social behavior*, which is more advanced action, as social behavior is behavior specifically directed at other people. The acceptability of behavior is evaluated relative to *social norms* and regulated by various *means* of *social control*.

Human behavior is an important factor in human society. According to Humanism, each human have a different behavior.

Factors affecting human behavior

- *Genetics*
- *Attitude* – It is the degree to which the person has a favourable or unfavourable evaluation of the behaviour in question.

- *Social Norms* – This is the influence of social pressure that is perceived by the individual (normative beliefs) to perform or not perform a certain behaviour.
- *Perceived Behavioural Control* – This is the individual's belief concerning how easy or difficult performing the behaviour will be.

From early psychology in the 19th century, the behaviorist school of thought ran concurrently and shared commonalities with the *psychoanalytic* and *Gestalt* movements in psychology into the 20th century; but also differed from the *mental philosophy* of the Gestalt psychologists in critical ways. Its main influences were *Ivan Pavlov*, who investigated *classical conditioning*, *Edward Lee Thorndike*, *John B. Watson* who rejected *introspective methods* and sought to restrict psychology to *experimental methods*, and *B.F. Skinner* who conducted research on *operant conditioning*. In the second half of the twentieth century, behaviorism was largely eclipsed as a result of the *cognitive revolution*.

A common theoretical base – most commonly called Social Learning theory, also known as Behaviour Modification, behavior therapy and cybernetics – guides this model. The stance taken here is that human beings are self-correction communication systems that modify behavior in response to information about how successfully tasks are navigated. For example: imagine a human being climbing a ladder in the dark. The first steps are tentative as the foot reaches for the treads. If the stride is too high, feedback is received as the foot encounters air and as to descend to make contact with the surface. If the step is too low, feedback results as the foot hits the riser. Gradually behavior is adjusted in accordance with the feedback until progress up the stairs is relatively comfortable.

Behavior model has its origin in the classical conditioning experiments of Pavlov (1972), the work of Thorndike (1911, 1913), on reward learning, and the study of Watson (1921) who applied Pavlovian principles to the psychological disorders of human beings.

Capitalizing on knowledge about how people respond to tasks and feedback, psychologists like Skinner have learned how to organize tasks and feedback structures to make it easy for human beings' self correcting capabilities to function.

Object orientation focuses on how data and behavior relate under a single class. Emphasis on the object naturally obscured how objects are associated and how their behavior is defined in detail. A previous series of articles addressed a more complete model of associations.

Behavior modeling was developed, for the most part, independently of object orientation. Consequently it is beneficial to review the three traditional categories of behavior model, examine how they differ, and explore how they can be used in an object-oriented way.

The behavior models above can be unified into one, but at the expense of making them more cumbersome to use.

An advanced technique to make a behavior model object-oriented is to associate each step with the changes to objects that the step is intended to cause, and associate those changes with the steps that they initiate. For example, the effects of fixing a roof, namely, a fixed roof and workers available for another job. Each has their own effect, billing the customer and assigning workers, respectively.

As a result Behavioral model in HRD includes programs for reducing phobias, developing social and athletic skills, replacing anxiety with relaxation, and learning the complexes of intellectual, social and physical skills to work in an organization and live a quality work life and also quality life. This model concentrates on observable behavior and clearly defined tasks and methods of communicating progress to the employee. It is based on a firm research foundation. This model is appropriate for personnel of all cadres and for an impressive number of objectives.

Simulations are used in this model. Simulations are constructed from descriptions of real life situations. A less-than-real-life environment is created. The employee engages in the activity to achieve the goal of the simulation and has to deal with realistic factors until goal is mastered.

CAREER DEVELOPMENT IN HRD

Many employees desire a career not just 'a job'. A career has been defined as the evolving sequence of a person's experiences over time. It is viewed fundamentally as a relationship between one (or more) organization(s) and the individual. To some a career is carefully worked out plan for self-advancement; to others it is a calling- a life role; to others it is a voyage of self-discovery and to still others it is life itself.

A career development system is a formal, organized, planned effort to achieve a balance between individual career needs and organizational workforce requirements. It is a mechanism for meeting the present and future human resource needs of an organization. Basically career development practices are designed to enhance the career satisfaction the career satisfaction of employees and to improve organizational effectiveness.

The future for people of HRD is full of opportunities. The future is going to be bright for genuine HRD managers. Those HRD managers who have entrepreneurial spirit, innovativeness and leadership qualities have a bright future for their career in HRD.

Responsibilities in Career Development

There are three key players who share responsibility for an employee's career development; the employee, the organization and the manager. Primary responsibility for an employee's career lies with the employee himself, but managers and the organizations can provide vita assistance. Management support is needed to establish a climate that fosters career development. It is very important that supervisors be involved in career development programmes.

The organizations responsibilities are:

- Providing resources for self-understanding and goal setting
- Setting and communicating missions, policies, goals and objectives
- Providing information on organization's options and career paths
- Providing raining, education and mobility opportunities
- Reinforcing and supporting the manager's role in career development and counseling

The manager's responsibilities are:

- Giving clear feedback about what employees should reasonably expect
- Providing forums for discussions
- Identifying employee potential
- Providing growth opportunities consistent with employee and organization goals
- Communicating the formal and informal realities of the organization
- Providing exposure for employees
- Linking employees to appropriate resources and people

The employee's responsibilities are:

- Self assessment
- Setting goals and plans
- Expressing expectations
- Making use of opportunities, education and training

Many organizations do not provide enough training to their current workforce. Many may not even have an adequate knowledge of their employees skill and talents. Organizations must figure out ways to create and environment that is more adaptive, collaborative and skill-ready.

It is said that working in an HRD department presents a unique opportunity to be a future CEO of the organization. There are great opportunities to HR managers to make an impact since challenges faced by organizations are HR challenge too. Recently and in future, HRD managers have openings as CLMs (Chief Learning Mangers) and CKMs (Chief Knowledge Managers). Other titles like managing partner of knowledge management, Knowledge Coordinator, Director of knowledge management, knowledge facilitator, knowledge leader, KM consultant, learning coordinator, learning specialist, organizational architect, director of organizational effectiveness, Vice president Knowledge Management are also used.

It is estimated that KM is a $ 7.2 billion market in the US. KM involves getting people to disseminate best practices, measuring

Table 6.1: Stages, Issues and Tasks of the Career Cycle of HRD

Stages	Issues	Specific Tasks
Growth, fantasy, exploration	Developing a basis for making realistic vocational choices. Obtaining education or training	Developing and discovering one's own needs and interests Getting maximum career information
Entry into world of work	Becoming a member of an organization or occupation	Learning how to liook for and secure a job
Basic training	Becoming an effective member quickly	Overcoming the insecurity of inexperience Learning to get along with superiors and co-workers
Full membership, in early career	Accepting the responsibility and discharging duties Developing and displaying social skills	Performing effectively Accepting subordinate status Developing initiative and and realistic expectations
Full membership, mid-career	Choosing a speciality Remaining technically competent Establishing a clear identity	Gaining a measure of independence Assessing own motives, talents Assessing organizational and occupational opportunities
Mid-career crisis	Reassessing own progress relative to ambitions Deciding relative importance of work and family	Becoming aware of career anchor Making specific choices about the present and future
Late career in non-leadership role	Becoming a mentor Broadening interests Deepening skills	Remaining technically competent Developing interpersonal skills Developing with younger persons
Late career in leadership role	Using skills and talents for organization's welfare Selecting and developing subordinates	Becoming more responsible for organization Handling power Balance career and family
Decline and disengagement	Learning to accept reduced power and responsibility	Finding new sources of satisfaction
Retirement	Adjusting to more drastic life style changes	Maintaining a sense of identity and self-worth without job

results, Performance Technology (PT), KM and HR professionals seem to be in synergistic roles. HRD managers can be of four different types:

- Future CEOs and CAs
- HRD Specialists

- Personnel specialists
- Sub-systems managers.

Career development in HRD is that organizations must now recognize and address if they hope to find and retain HRD employees who will help them meet their constantly shifting demands. It is high time that HRD managers be looked on for promoting learning and competence building.

INTEGRATED HRD SYSTEMS

HRD System

A system has certain characteristics. It has an input, output and a process. It has components and elements that make it a system. A system helps in planning. It brings about predictability, discipline, and security. A system is a planned way of making things happen. A system has its own objectives, components or elements and a process. The purpose of any HRD system is broadly to build the competencies and / or commitment of individuals, dyads, teams and the entire organization through various techniques. Its objective is to build a lasting culture so that employees earn and give their best in a continuous way. The techniques available for an organization are put into sub-systems and become HRD systems or sub-systems. The following are the techniques that are available and have been considered to be the sub-systems:

1. Induction Training
2. training
3. performance planning
4. performance analysis and review
5. performance development
6. performance counseling
7. performance appraisals
8. rewards and recognition
9. potential appraisal and development
10. career paths, career planning and development
11. job rotation

12. quality circles and other team – based activities
13. communications
14. organizational diagnosis and development (OD interventions)
15. team building, role clarity and other mechanisms

These subsystems get propagated to ensure the maximum level of achievement of HRD goals. Some of them get grouped either for administrative convenience or in order to ensure synergy in terms of the value. For example, induction training and training are normally grouped to form the training system. The training system attempts to ensure that the technique of training is used effectively, efficiently, appropriately and not misused. It becomes a system by formulating its own objectives, elements inputs, output and process. The output of systems, subsystem that link it to other subsystem.

For example: the objectives of the training subsystem could be the following:

- To ensure that technical, managerial, human and conceptual competencies are developed in the employees on a continuous basis so as to enable them to perform their current jobs effectively and also to get them ready to perform the new jobs as they come.
- To offer the necessary competency building inputs to all employees in a systematic, scientific and efficient way
- To offer the required value and attitude –based training to ensure that a lasting and self-sustaining culture is built in the organization.

The inputs for the training system could be the following:

- Training needs identified on the basis of performance gaps in the previous year, performance opportunities for the next year. These are assessed through performance appraisals and come as inputs to the training sub-system.
- Training needs assessed on the basis of technological changes in the organization, strategic moves and other changes in the environment
- Training needs assessed on the basis of the norms, values and other cultural aspects the organization wants to develop in its members.

The outputs expected could be defined in terms of the following:

- New competencies acquired by the employee
- New competencies acquired by dyads, teams and the organization as a whole.

These new competencies will become inputs for improved performance, cost reduction, speed, efficiency and quality improvement in products or processes.

The **elements** of training sub-system may include the following:

- Methods of identifying training needs: performance appraisals. Training needs identification surveys, organizational diagnosis surveys, etc.
- Training department
- Training managers or the HRD staff handling the training sub-system and their own competencies
- Faculty and other competencies
- Training methods used and strategies used
- Trainers and their competencies
- Training evaluation methods

There could be several other elements and each of the above can further be broken into elements.

The **processes** deal essentially with the organization of the above elements and the rules, procedures and steps that govern the use of the above elements. For example

- Method of determining training needs
- The timing
- Method of using training needs to prepare training plans, etc.
- Methods of sponsoring the employee for training
- Pre-training preparation required
- Process of conducting the training
- Process of evaluating it
- Follow-up methods, etc.

This rationale is followed for all the sub-systems of HRD.

Basic Assumptions underlying HRD systems are:

- HRD system is a subsystem of a larger system (organization)
- HRD system is an organic whole: all the parts are interlinked
- The main task of HRD system is to develop enabling capabilities (proacting role)
- All managers share the responsibility of human resource management
- The responsibilities of HRD system relate to people, systems, and the process of the total organization.
- The major attention of HRD system is on developing people and their competencies.
- HRD systems and procedures should be designed on the basis of process values to reduce human wastage
- People are primarily motivated by challenges and opportunities for development and creativity.

A number of Human Resource Development frameworks are being used to improve the HRD systems in India. An Integrated Systems Approach was evolved for Indian organizations at the Indian Institute of Management, Ahmedabad by Pareek and Rao (1975, 1977).

Integrated HRD Systems

An integrated system approach was evolved for Indian organizations at the Indian Institute of Management, Ahmedabad by Pareek and Rao. This system envisages a separated HRD department for effective designing and implementation of HRD systems. It envisaged strategy as a starting point; and therefore focused on all the systems to achieve organizational goals and employee satisfaction. It aimed at synergy, proposed the phased evolution of HRD function and included most of the elements of the Human Capital Approach.

This system has the following elements:

1. a separate and differentiated HR department with full time HRD staff

2. 6 HRD subsystems including OD
3. inter-linkages between the various sub-systems.
4. designed with 14 principles
5. linked to other subsystems of Human Resource Function

In the beginning L&T, SBI and its associates are using the Integrated HRD systems approach and have created a new HR department. By the mid-80's a large number of organizations in India have established HR departments on these lines.

HRD AND MANAGEMENT

Getting things done through people and other resources to accomplish leadership, and decide how to use organizational resources and providing direction and leadership are what managers do. Management is considered to be universal because it uses organizational resources to accomplish goals and attain high performance in all types of profit and non-profit organizations.

Mary Parker Follett (1868–1933), who wrote on the topic in the early twentieth century, defined management as "the art of getting things done through people". She also described management as philosophy. One can also think of management functionally, as the action of measuring a quantity on a regular basis and of adjusting some initial *plan*; or as the actions taken to reach one's intended *goal*. This applies even in situations where planning does not take place. From this perspective, Frenchman *Henri Fayol* considers management to consist of seven *functions*:

1. *planning*
2. *organizing*
3. *leading*
4. *co-ordinating*
5. *controlling*
6. *staffing*
7. *motivating*

Some people, however, find this definition, while useful, far too narrow. The phrase "management is what managers do" occurs widely, suggesting the difficulty of defining management, the shifting nature of definitions, and the connection of managerial practices with the existence of a managerial *cadre* or *class*.

Some definitions of management are:

- Organization and coordination of the activities of an enterprise in accordance with certain policies and in achievement of clearly defined objectives. Management is often included as a factor of production along with machines, materials, and money.
- According to the management guru Peter Drucker (1909–2005), the basic task of a management is twofold: marketing and innovation. Practice of modern management owes its origin to the 16th century enquiry into low-efficiency and failures of certain enterprises, conducted by the English statesman Sir Thomas More (1478–1535).
- Directors and managers who have the power and responsibility to make decisions to manage an enterprise. As a discipline, management comprises the interlocking functions of formulating corporate policy and organizing, planning, controlling, and directing the firm's resources to achieve the policy's objectives. The size of management can range from one person in a small firm to hundreds or thousands of managers in multinational companies. In large firms the board of directors formulates the policy which is implemented by the chief executive officer.

"Management is the attainment of organizational goals in an effective and efficient manner through planning, organizing, leading and controlling organizational resources."

Managers use a multitude of skills to perform these two functions of management i.e.,

1. The four functions planning, organizing, leading and controlling
2. The attainment of organizational goals in an effective and efficient manner.

Management theorists identify additional management functions, such as, staffing, communication, or decision making.

Planning: means defining goals for future organizational performance and deciding on the tasks and use of resources needed to attain them. A lack of planning or poor planning can hurt an organization's performance.

Organizing: typically follows planning and reflects how the organization tries to accomplish the plan. Organizing involves the assignment of tasks, the grouping of tasks into departments, and the allocation of resources too departments.

Leading: Providing leadership is a very important management function. Leading is the use of influence to motivate employees to achieve organizational goals. Leading means creating a shared culture and values, communicating goals to employees throughout the organization and infusing employees with a desire to perform at a higher level. In an era of international competition, the ability to shape culture, communicate goals, and motivate employees is critical to business success.

Controlling: it is monitoring employee's activities, determining whether the organization is on target toward its goals, and making corrections as necessary. Managers must ensure that the organization is moving towards its goal.

HRD AND MANAGEMENT

Quality is a key to achieve excellence in management which includes functions such as finance, human resource, materials and scheduling. Conventional management system focused on each of these identities independently. Modern management insisted on higher effectiveness. Hence strategies such as Total Quality Management were introduced. Total Quality management is a management philosophy where every individual in an organization is motivated to work towards a common vision, in an ideal environment, continuously improving their performance, resulting in better business opportunities.

Management for TQM

HRM seeks to build and maintain an environment for quality excellence to better enable the work force to achieve the company's quality and operational performance objectives. In TQ organizations,

HRM units develop policies and procedures to ensure that employees can perform multiple roles, improvise when necessary and direct themselves towards continuous improvement of both product quality and customer service. The people structure has been changed to achieve quality in work place.

Branches of management theory also exist relating to *non-profits* and to government: such as *public administration*, *public management*, and educational management. Further, management programs related to *civil-society* organizations have also spawned programs in *nonprofit management* and *social entrepreneurship*.

All policies must be discussed with all managerial personnel and staff that is required in the execution of any departmental policy.

- Organizational change is strategically achieved through the implementation of the eight-step plan of action established by John P. Kotter: Increase urgency, get the vision right, communicate the buy-in, empower action, create short-term wins, don't let up, and make change stick.

Top-level management

- Require an extensive knowledge of management roles and skills.
- They have to be very aware of external factors such as markets.
- Their decisions are generally of a long-term nature
- Their decisions are made using analytic, directive, conceptual and/or behavioral/participative processes
- They are responsible for **strategic** decisions.
- They have to chalk out the plan and see that plan may be effective in the future.
- They are executive in nature.

Middle management

- Mid-level managers have a specialized understanding of certain managerial tasks.
- They are responsible for carrying out the decisions made by top-level management.

Lower management

- This level of management ensures that the decisions and plans taken by the other two are carried out.
- Lower-level managers' decisions are generally short-term ones.

Foreman/lead hand

- They are people who have direct supervision over the working force in office factory, sales field or other workgroup or areas of activity.

Rank and File

- The responsibilities of the persons belonging to this group are even more restricted and more specific than those of the foreman.

Public, private, and voluntary sectors place different demands on managers, but all must retain the faith of those who select them (if they wish to retain their jobs), retain the faith of those people that fund the organization, and retain the faith of those who work for the organization. If they fail to convince employees of the advantages of staying rather than leaving, they may tip the organization into a downward spiral of hiring, training, firing, and recruiting. Management also has the task of *innovating* and of improving the functioning of organizations.

Towards the end of the 20th century, business management came to consist of six separate branches, namely:

- *Human resource* management
- *Operations management* or production management
- *Strategic management*
- *Marketing management*
- *Financial management*
- *Information technology management* responsible for management information systems

In the 21st century observers find it increasingly difficult to subdivide management into functional categories in this way. More and more processes simultaneously involve several categories. Instead, one tends to think in terms of the various processes, tasks, and objects subject to management.

The Human Resources Management (HRM) function includes a variety of activities, and key among them is deciding what staffing needs you have and whether to use independent contractors or hire employees to fill these needs, recruiting and training the best employees, ensuring they are high performers, dealing with performance issues, and ensuring your personnel and management practices conform to various regulations. Activities also include managing your approach to employee benefits and compensation, employee records and personnel policies. Usually small businesses (for-profit or nonprofit) have to carry out these activities themselves because they can't yet afford part- or full-time help. However, they should always ensure that employees have — and are aware of — personnel policies which conform to current regulations. These policies are often in the form of employee manuals, which all employees have.

Note that some people distinguish a difference between between HRM (a major management activity) and HRD (Human Resource Development, a profession). Those people might include HRM in HRD, explaining that HRD includes the broader range of activities to develop personnel inside of organizations, including, e.g., career development, training, organization development, etc.

There is a long-standing argument about where HR-related functions should be organized into large organizations, e.g., "should HR be in the Organization Development department or the other way around?"

More recently, organizations consider the "HR Department" as playing a major role in staffing, training and helping to manage people so that people and the organization are performing at maximum capability in a highly fulfilling manner which is vital importance for the management.

BARRIERS TO HRD

Human resource development faces significant barriers. They may be:

- HR practitioners are perceived as experts in handling HR matters, but are not experts in managing organizations

- Financial matters often take precedence over Human resource development
- Conflict may exist between short term and long term HR needs.
- Conflict exists between qualitative and quantitative approaches to HRD.
- Non-involvement of operating administrators renders HRD ineffective. HRD is not strictly within the domain of HR department. Successful HRD needs a coordinated effort on the part of administrators, managers and HR specialists.

It is commonly observed that "knowledge is power". Conversely, lack of knowledge is often a weakness, rendering those without the information less able to take advantage of opportunities and rendering them more vulnerable. This is particularly important with respect to HRD. Education also undoubtedly plays an important part in the filtering of information and the interpretation and expression.

Economic barriers: costs and affordability

Costs are generally perceived to be the greatest barrier to HRD. Organizations and People may simply not be able to afford the HRD services, especially the poor in developing countries. However, their readiness and ability to absorb ongoing costs such as those associated with education, and especially secondary and tertiary education and professional training, may be much less.

Geographical barriers

Geographical distance is readily recognized as a barrier, but its effects are neither consistent from one society to another nor uniform within the society. The concepts of distance and mobility become crucial.

Administrative barriers

HRD requires a certain amount of administrative formality. Lack of education or illiteracy, as well as a lack of access to technology, can be cross-cutting issues that act on their own, or compound other barriers to HRD. Administrative impediments have long been recognized as one set of barriers to HRD. These may be formalized in the specific administrative structure of HRD

Social and other barriers

There are numerous social barriers to HRD. These can be considered at the individual or family level and also at the societal level. At the individual or household level, age, gender, income, education and health status all come into play in influencing who will use certain services of HRD and how often. Evidence is not clear even with respect to the same types of service. For example, gender has been found in different country settings to increase or decrease the effectiveness of HRD. Much is dependent on additional factors such as costs and cultural norms. An important concept of equity must be considered in this context.

Three groupings of determinants are often identified in psychosocial studies: (a) needs; (b) abilities; and (c) opportunities.

The HRD practices are in part influenced by such characteristics as age, income, educational level, phase of life and household situation. They are also heavily influenced by health status. Abilities can also affects HRD practices. Cognitive, sensory, intellectual or physical abilities influence HRD.

Lack of knowledge (and literacy) can be a potent barrier to the use of HRD services. Once illiterate or with limited functional literacy, people may be unable to use HRD services.

At the aggregate level, religious and cultural barriers too act on HRD.

Conflict

A further group of barriers to HRD, stem from conflicts in the organization.

HRD: FOR SOCIAL CHANGE

Social change is a general term which refers to:

- change in *social structure*: the *nature*, the *social institutions*, the *social behaviour* or the *social relations* of a *society*, *community* of people, and so on.
- When behaviour pattern changes, in large numbers and is visible and sustained it results in a social change. Once there is a

deviance from culturally inherited values, it may result in a rebe l llion against the established system, causing a change in the social order.

- Any event or action that affects a group of individuals that have shared values or characteristics.
- Acts of *advocacy* for the *cause* of changing *society* in a normative way (subjective).

To make the concept of social change more clear, we are giving some definitions as under:

(1) "Social changes are a term used to describe variation in or modification of any aspects of social processes, social interaction or social organization." -Sir Jones

(2) "Social changes are variations from the accepted modes of life whether due to alterations in geographic conditions, in cultural equipment, composition of the population or ideologies and whether brought about by diffusion or invention with in the group."--Gillin and Gillin

(3) "Social change means that large number of persons is engaged in activities that differ from those in which they or their immediate fore-fathers were engaged in some time before. Society is composed of a vast and complex network of patterned relationship, in which all men participate, when human behaviour is in the process of modification that is only another way of indicating that social change is occurring."

There is difference of opinion among scholars about the nature and form of social change. In this connection the views of some famous sociologists namely; Brown, Chopin, Spencer, Lister Ward and Ogburn are as under:

(1) According to Brown, there is no difference between social change and cultural change. Both are interrelated in the sense that cultural change is an important part of social change.

(2) Chopin has divided cultural changes in to three categories - (i) Those changes which are concerned with material culture; (ii) Those changes which are connected with non material culture; and (iii) Those changes which are linked up with composite

culture. The examples of these three are serially social order, ideals, and forms of administration.

(3) According to Spencer, social change and social evaluation are identical. In his opinion social changes are uniform, gradual and progressive. Spencer has further pointed out that as we progress from less painful position to more comfortable positions, the process of social changes also undergoes the essential stages of evaluation.

(4) Lister ward does not agree with the views of Spencer. According to him, social change is related to the changes in social aims and aspirations of individuals. Hence, it is not based on the principle of evaluation but is planned, intelligent and purposive. Each human being determines those aims according to his intelligence, which he can achieve and this achievement brings about social change.

(5) According to Ogburn, there is no distinction between social change and cultural change. He advocates two forms of culture namely - (i) Material, and (ii) non- material. Material culture is concerned with all those things and objects which man has made for his welfare and happiness. Radio, television, means of transport and communication etc., are examples in this connection. Non-material culture is concerned with human ideas, attitudes, values, habits, customs, traditions and our mentalities.

Ogburn asserts that first the change occurs in the material culture and then in the non-material. When material culture changes and non-material remains the same or lags behind, cultural lag occurs. Indian society is an example of cultural lag. Education is the only means to remove this cultural lag.

The term is used in the study of *history*, *sociology*, economies, and *politics*, and includes topics such as the success or failure of different political systems, *globalization*, *democratization*, development and *economic growth*. The term can encompass concepts as broad as *revolution* and *paradigm shift*, to narrow changes such as a particular cause within small town government. The concept of social change imply measurement of some characteristics of this group of individuals. While the term is usually applied to changes that are beneficial to society, it may result in negative side-effects or consequences that undermine or eliminate existing ways of life that are considered positive.

Models of Social Change

- Hegelian— The classic *Hegelian* dialectic model of change is based on the interaction of opposing forces. Starting from a point of momentary stasis, Thesis countered by Antithesis first yields conflict but subsequently results in a new Synthesis.
- Kuhnian— *Thomas Kuhn* in *The Structure of Scientific Revolutions* argued with respect to the *Copernican* Revolution that people are unlikely to jettison an unworkable paradigm, despite many indications that the paradigm is not functioning properly, until a better paradigm can be presented.
- Heraclitan— The Greek philosopher *Heraclitus* used the metaphor of a river to speak of change thus, "On those stepping into rivers staying the same other and other waters flow." (DK22B12) What Heraclitus seems to be suggesting here, later interpretations notwithstanding, is that in order for the river to remain the river change must constantly be taking place. Thus one may think of the Heraclitan model as parallel to that of a living organism, which, in order to remain alive must constantly be changing.
- Daoist—The Chinese philosophical work *Dao De Jing*, I.8 and II.78 uses the metaphor of water as the ideal agent of change. Water, though soft and yielding, will eventually wear away stone. Change in this model is to be natural, harmonius, and steady, though imperceptible.

SOCIAL CHANGE AND HRD

Social change means change in the structure and functions of human society. The human life is not static. It is under constant change in the ideals, attitudes and values of an individual which affects social attributes and social structure, which no society in the world can escape.

HR specialists can help in removing the factors that resist social change. The factors that could resist culture change are:

- Cultural inertia
- Fear of new things
- Vested interests
- Degree of isolation

Few factors which promote social change are promoted by HR specialists. They are :

- The physical environment
- Scientific inventions and researches
- Interdynamics.

HR personnel could be used by government and societies. They should be agents of change in society and may take care to prevent crime, counseling centres, initiate change, use media to bring about change, etc. They take up researches to find reasons behind increasing crime rates, pathology etc., in the society and suggest methods to contain the same. They should be able to work with newspapers and media and influence society. They should be attached to the media and other agencies. They could propagate ideas which promote social change in all fields of life. They help in bring about social change since they

- Perpetualize eternal values
- Promote capacity to welcome and accept social change
- Evaluate social change
- Aid the coming of the new social change
- Promote Transmission of culture
- Promote unity and total integrity
- Maintain human and social relations
- Educate about social change
- Increase the areas of knowledge
- Provide leadership role for social changes.

Modernization results in social change. Modernization is a concept symbolizing a movement of progressive thinking, evolution of better techniques of production and scientific advancement with the main objective of removing blind beliefs, destructive attitudes worthless faiths in order to achieve a modern progressive society. HRD could act as a vehicle to equip the citizens with the necessary insight, capacity and intelligence to achieve all kinds of scientific areas of human activity.

Research and campaign designing etc., are their core competencies of HR professionals which could be utilized for bringing about smooth and constructive social change.

SUMMARY

Behavior modeling was developed, for the most part, independently of object orientation. Consequently it is beneficial to review the three traditional categories of behavior model, examine how they differ, and explore how they can be used in an object-oriented way. The behavior models above can be unified into one, but at the expense of making them more cumbersome to use. A career development system is a formal, organized, planned effort to achieve a balance between individual career needs and organizational workforce requirements. It is a mechanism for meeting the present and future human resource needs of an organization. Basically career development practices are designed to enhance the career satisfaction the career satisfaction of employees and to improve organizational effectiveness.

An integrated system approach was evolved for Indian organizations at the Indian Institute of Management, Ahmedabad by Pareek and Rao. This system envisages a separated HRD department for effective designing and implementation of HRD systems. It envisaged strategy as a starting point; and therefore focused on all the systems to achieve organizational goals and employee satisfaction. It aimed at synergy, proposed the phased evolution of HRD function and included most of the elements of the Human Capital Approach.

UNIT 7

RESEARCH AND DEVELOPMENT IN HUMAN RESOURCE DEVELOPMENT

INTRODUCTION

Scientific research is the systematic investigation of hypothesized proposition about the relationship among natural phenomena. Its purpose is to generate knowledge and further the field of a profession. Research in HRD aims at identifying a problem, generating alternatives and solving it. Research in HRD has the task of searching for, and analyzing, facts to the end that human resource problems may be solved or principles and laws governing their solution derived.

It involves the systematic study of human resources for the purpose of maximizing personal and organizational goal achievement. The three important research methods are the case study, the survey and the experiment.

Case Study: A case is an in-depth analysis of a single setting. This design is frequently used when a little is known about the phenomena being studied and the researcher wants to look at relevant concepts intensively and thoroughly. A variety of methods are used to gather information, including interviews, questionnaires and personal observation.

When the researcher is to uncover the underlying reason for occurrence of a problem the case study is often used. By using this method, the researcher can identify causes of specific problems, typical problems for which case study might be used include identifying the reason for an excessively high turnover at a particular plant; a high absenteeism rate in a specific department, a high accident rate at a certain construction site, low morale in a particular department, the underlying reasons for a strike ate a particular section.

The Field Survey: A field survey usually relies on a questionnaire distributed to a sample of people chosen from a larger population. Field surveys provide information about a much larger segment of the population than case studies. They also provide an abundant data in quantifiable form, which facilitates statistical analysis and the compilation of normative data for comparative purposes.

A major function of human resource research is to periodically check the pulse of the organization to determine the employees attitude toward other people, and attitudes to such factors as job satisfaction, pay, commitment to the organization, and supervision. The primary tool for the researcher in this endeavor is often attitude survey, which is also known as the opinion survey.

Laboratory Experiment: is a method of inquiry which certain variables being manipulated while others are held constant and their effect is being studied on certain variables. With this method, there is both a control group and an experimental group. The control group remains constant and operate as it did under the old environment whereas selected variables are manipulated within the experimental group. For instance, the researcher may desire to determine the effect of a new training programme on productivity. The control group would continue to perform tasks in the conventional manner. The experimental group would receive the training and it is assumed that if a change in productivity occurs it would have been because of the training.

Field Experiment: a field experiment is similar to a laboratory experiment except that it is conducted in a real organization. The organization setting provides greater realism, making generalization to other organizational situation more valid.

The following articles published in the *Human Resources Development Quarterly* 1999 issues 23 is indicative of the kind of research trends followed in the USD:

- Formal development relation: a survey of organizational practices
- Integration learning with working: a re-conception of the role of the work place in learning

- Formal mentoring as a strategy of Human Resource Development
- Managers as Facilitators of learning in learning organizations
- Field investigation of the relationship among adult curiosity, work place learning and job performance
- Managing the HRD function and service quality: a call for a new approach
- Learning and performance; just the end of the beginning
- Developing of a generalized learning transfer system inventory
- Developing from job experiences

Research from across the world in the last few years has shown that good HR practices and policies can go a long way in influencing organizational growth and development. Research has shown that the following are some HR practices that effective firms adopt with people:

- Financial incentives for excellent performance
- Work organization practices that motivate employee effort and capture the benefits of know-how and skill
- Rigorous selection and selectivity in recruitment
- Higher than average wages
- Employee share ownership plans
- Extensive information sharing
- Decentralization of decision-making and empowerment
- Work organization based on self managing teams
- High investment in training and skill development
- Having people do multiple jobs and job-rotation
- Elimination of status symbols
- A more compressed distribution of salaries across and within levels
- Promotion from within
- A long-term perspective
- Measurement of HR practices and policy implementation
- A coherent view of employment relations.

Arthur Yeung and Bob Berman (1997) point out that HR practices can play three major roles:

1. Building critical organizational capabilities
2. Enhancing employee satisfaction
3. Improving customer and shareholder satisfaction.

Research studies have indicated that a large number of articles in professional journals are research-based. The journal *Advances in developing Human Resources* of AHRD has published 6 issues so far; each of them devoted to a special theme. The themes are also indicative of the contemporary concerns of HRD professionals.

1. Performance Improvement: Theory and Practice
2. Action Learning: Successful strategies for Team and Organization Development
3. Informal Learning on the Job
4. Developing Human Resources for the Global Economy.
5. Strategic Perspectives on Knowledge, Competence and Expertise
6. Developing High Performance Leadership Competency.

In the US alone, over 1000 scholars are enrolled for their doctoral programs and several hundreds of professors undertake academic research. HRD professionals and leading institutes of managements are taking active interest in HR-related research. IIM, Ahmedabad, Bangalore, Lucknow and Kolkata have promoted research in HRD. IITs have also started PhDs programs in management and human resource management. Institutions like the Academy of HRD, Ahmedabad has its unique Fellow program in HRD, in collaboration with XLRI, Jamshedpur. The AHRD-XLRI has produced 8 Fellows in the first 7 years of their collaboration. Universities and private institutes are also promoting research in HRD.

"HRD is a process by which the employees of an organization are helped, in a continuous, planned way, to acquire or sharpen capabilities required to perform various functions associated with their present or expected future roles; required to perform various functions associated with their present or expected future roles; develop their general capabilities as individuals and discover and exploit their own inner potential for their own and/or organizational development purposes; develop an organizational culture in which the supervisor-subordinate relationships, teamwork and collaboration among sub-units are strong and contribute to the professional well being, motivation and pride of employees".

Rao (1985)

During the last decade or so, a lot has been talked, written and experimented on Research and development organizations in India. Various seminars and conferences have been conducted to bring about its awareness and appreciations in the development sector. However, it is seen that there is lack of clarity about its role and importance in the development of the social and economical conditions of the nation. Hence this unit introduces you to HRD in Research and development organizations, the different developmental needs in research and development like Creativity, Attitudes, Communication, Interpersonal Relationship, Team Building, Leadership, and Motivation and the various approaches to HRD.

HRD IN RESEARCH AND DEVELOPMENT ORGANIZATIONS

There is no doubt that HRD has a tremendous influence on the outcomes of Research and Development organizations. There is ample research and experimental data to suggest this. HRD simply means competence building, commitment building and culture building. Without competencies many tasks of the organization many not be completed cost-effectively or with optimal efficiency. Without commitment, they may not be done at all or may be done at such a slow pace that they lose relevance. Without appropriate culture the organization may not survive. These three Cs are very important to make any Research and Development Organization function effectively and efficiently. Hence HRD is very essential in Research and development organizations.

HRD in the context of research and development organizations is a process by which the employees of the organization are helped in a continuous, planned way to sharpen their capabilities.

Human Resource development can contribute a great deal in preparing individuals in Research and Development Organizations. In order for this to take place, it is vital that HRD is a part of any Research and Development Organizations. Swanson and Torraco (1995) emphasize that organizations must develop relevant expertise in order to realize the strategic advantage of human resources. Highly competent HRD professionals are needed to identify performance requirements that align with objectives and strategies of Research and Development organizations. At the individual level, HRD can focus on developing personnel throughout the organization.

DEVELOPMENTAL NEEDS IN RESEARCH AND DEVELOPMENT

In human resource development, factors other than those associated with functionality too matter. Those factors are the developmental needs in research and development. A few major developmental needs include Creativity, Attitudes, Communication, Interpersonal Relationship, Team Building, Leadership, and Motivation. Let us look at each of them in detail.

CREATIVITY

"Only dead fish swim with the stream". Living individuals are creative and dare to swim against and look for different ways of doing things. It is such live and creative people who contribute and are wanted for the development of the organization and for the society as a whole.

If Human Resource Development is to fulfill the hopes of those who believe it is an essential contributor to social and economic success then there are many challenges to be met. Among these are the challenges raised by the growth of the creative class, with creative and cultural industries now forming a major sector of employment and creativity, individuality and imagination being highly valued in the workplace. The Challenges of Human Resources Development questions how the increasing importance of creativity impacts on the ways in which we understand HRD, and what its role is in Research and development.

Creativity has become a valued commodity in the world. Fostering creativity in the workplace contributes significantly to peak performance, a creative approach to problem solving, and effective teamwork. Fostering creativity in the workplace contributes significantly to peak performance, a creative approach to problem solving, and effective teamwork.

Improvement in work results in a research and development organization is possible when employees,

- Cultivate creativity in themselves and others
- Discover ways to encourage creative thinking in themselves and others
- Create environments conducive for creative change
- Use creative thinking processes for making decisions
- Utilize humor to generate creativity
- Build the morale of others by empowering them to contribute their creative ideas
- Discover ways to use your creative ideas to foster fun and productive work environment

Lynne Levesque shows that creativity, like intelligences, exists in a variety of forms, and demonstrates that high-performance organizations need to make use of creativity in all its dimensions. It takes more than just "thinking outside the box" to build a flexible, adaptive organization that will survive competitive battles, grow and prosper, and provide the environment that attracts and keeps its best talent. On the basis of her research in personality, innovation, and creativity, as well as her experience helping top executives achieve their full potential. Levesque describes eight distinct creative talents. People of each talent have a unique way of looking at challenges, collecting data, and generating creative solutions. Each individual involved in research and development has to discover his own creative talents and use them to further his professional and personal lives.

Creativity is an area of academic investigation that is of growing importance, with a need for researchers and practitioners, specifically in HRD, to have theories and models that offer sound guidance for the creative journey. HRD can take an active role in innovation. As the organizational landscape becomes more unpredictable and complex, and as the rate of change continues to increase, creativity is becoming more and more vital to organizational success and survival. Human resource development (HRD) should be a primary player in the creative process because human capability and expertise are needed in order to successfully navigate the journey in the organization.

HRD is recognized as a key component in improving innovation efforts. HRD should strive to better understand exactly how innovation efforts can succeed. HRD helps in building human capacity, and developing organizational environments that are conducive to innovation. Creativity is of paramount importance to the innovation process. Therefore the findings of creativity research should be thoroughly considered in organizations where innovation processes are required. It signals the significance of exploring creativity and HRD by looking at knowledge workplaces, workforce projections, work values, occupation projections, on-the-job training, and entrepreneurship.

It has also been found that creativity and HRD have similar learning and performance variables. McLean (2005) pointed out that supports for creativity and innovation include organizational encouragement, supervisory encouragement, work group encouragement, freedom and autonomy, and resources. He also points out that the major impediment to creativity and innovation as evident in the literature is control. Then, underscoring the intimate relationship between creativity and innovation, McLean (2005) aptly notes that "creativity without innovation is of significantly diminished value" because it might not result in anything, and "innovation without creativity is an engine without any fuel". Finally, McLean (2005) suggests that HRD professionals can positively impact creativity, organizational culture, and climate through organization development (OD) and training and development (T&D) initiatives.

Training is described as "the process through which skills are developed, information is provided, and attributes are nurtured, in order to help individuals who work in organizations to become more effective and efficient in their work" (Davis & Davis, 1998). These practices take place at the individual, group, process, and organization levels, which provides a logical fit with the multilevel model presented in this paper. Training and development interventions can be specifically designed to build capacities that can enable individuals to improve creativity and thus innovation.

OD interventions can be designed to create an organizational environment that nurtures innovation. Organization development is defined as "the system-wide application of behavioral science knowledge to the planned development, improvement, and reinforcement of the strategies, structures, and processes that lead to organizational effectiveness" (Cummings & Worley, 2001).

Efforts should be made to develop creativity at all levels of the organization because this will drive innovation and allow individuals to respond to the changing organizational environment (Egan, 2005a). Van de Ven et al. (1999) stress that because the innovation journey is so complex, management cannot ensure success in the process, rather, management can influence the odds of success. There are many possible approaches managers can take to doing this – such as increasing their knowledge and understanding of the journey. The two roles identified for HRD in this process (the development of individual capacity as it relates to innovation and the creation of an organizational environment conducive to innovation) are aimed at increasing the odds of innovation success. More specifically, HRD can develop both the individual and the organization through various Training & Development processes and through Organizational Development efforts.

ATTITUDES

Attitude is a hypothetical construct that represents an individual's degree of like or dislike for an item. Attitudes are judgments. Attitudes are generally positive or negative views of a person, place, thing, or event. People can also be conflicted or ambivalent toward an object, meaning that they simultaneously possess both positive and negative attitudes toward the item in question.

Jung's definition of attitude is "a readiness of the *psyche* to act or react in a certain way".

Attitudes very often come in pairs, one conscious and the other unconscious. Within the broad definition Jung defines several attitudes.

The main attitude dualities that Jung defines are the following:

- *Consciousness and the unconscious*: The "presence of two attitudes is extremely frequent, one *conscious* and the other unconscious. This means that consciousness has a constellation of contents different from that of the unconscious, a duality particularly evident in *neurosis*" (Jung, [1921] 1971: par. 687).
- *Extraversion and introversion*: This pair is so elementary to Jung's theory of types that he labeled them the "attitude-types".
- *Rational and irrational attitudes*: "I conceive reason as an attitude" (Jung, [1921] 1971: par. 785).
- The rational attitude subdivides into the thinking and feeling psychological functions, each with its attitude.
- The irrational attitude subdivides into the sensing and intuition psychological functions, each with its attitude. "There is thus a typical thinking, feeling, sensation, and intuitive attitude" (Jung, [1921] 1971: par. 691).
- *Individual and social attitudes*: Many of the latter are "isms".

Attitudes develop on the **ABC** model (affect, behavior, and *cognition*). The affective response is an *emotional* response that expresses an individual's degree of preference for an entity. The behavioral intention is a verbal indication or typical behavioral tendency of an individual. The cognitive response is a cognitive evaluation of the entity that constitutes an individual's beliefs about the object. Most attitudes are the result of either direct experience or *observational learning* from the environment.

Unlike *personality*, attitudes are expected to change as a function of *experience*. Tesser (1993) has argued that hereditary variables may affect attitudes - but believes that they may do so indirectly. For example, if one inherits the disposition to become an extrovert, this may affect one's attitude to certain styles of music.

Attitudes can be changed through persuasion. The celebrated work of Carl Hovland, at Yale University in the 1950s and 1960s, helped to advance knowledge of persuasion. In Hovland's view, we should understand attitude change as a response to communication. He and his colleagues did experimental research into the factors that can affect the persuasiveness of a message:

1. *Target Characteristics*: These are characteristics that refer to the person who receives and processes a message. One such trait is intelligence - it seems that more intelligent people are less easily persuaded by one-sided messages. Another variable that has been studied in this category is self-esteem. Although it is sometimes thought that those higher in self-esteem are less easily persuaded, there is some evidence that the relationship between self-esteem and persuasibility is actually curvilinear, with people of moderate self-esteem being more easily persuaded than both those of high and low self-esteem levels (Rhodes & Woods, 1992). The mind frame and mood of the target also plays a role in this process.
2. *Source Characteristics:* The major source characteristics are expertise, trustworthiness and interpersonal attraction or attractiveness. The credibility of a perceived message has been found to be a key variable here (Hovland & Weiss, 1951); if one reads a report about health and believes it came from a professional medical journal, one may be more easily persuaded than if one believes it is from a popular newspaper. Some psychologists have debated whether this is a long-lasting effect and Hovland and Weiss (1951) found the effect of telling people that a message came from a credible source disappeared after several weeks (the so-called "sleeper effect"). Whether there is a sleeper effect is controversial. Received wisdom is that if people are informed of the source of a message before hearing it, there is less likelihood of a sleeper effect than if they are told a message and then told its source.
3. *Message Characteristics*: The nature of the message plays a role in persuasion. Sometimes presenting both sides of a story is useful to help change attitudes.

Cognitive Routes: A message can appeal to an individual's cognitive evaluation to help change an attitude. In the *central route* to persuasion the individual is presented with the data and motivated to evaluate the data and arrive at an attitude changing conclusion. In the *peripheral route* to attitude change, the individual is encouraged to not look at the content but at the source. This is commonly seen in modern advertisements that feature celebrities. In some cases, physician, doctors or experts are used. In other cases film stars are used for their attractiveness.

Emotion and Attitude Change

Emotion is a common component in *persuasion*, *social influence*, and *attitude change*. Much of attitude research emphasized the importance of affective or emotion components (Breckler & Wiggins, 1992). Emotion works hand-in-hand with the cognitive process, or the way we think, about an issue or situation. Emotional appeals are commonly found in advertising, health campaigns and political messages. Recent examples include no-smoking health campaigns and political campaign advertising emphasizing the fear of terrorism.

Taking into consideration current attitude research, Breckler and Wiggins (1992) define attitudes as "mental and neural representations, organized through experience, exerting a directive or dynamic influence on behavior" (p. 409).

Attitudes and attitude objects are functions of cognitive, affective and conative components. Attitudes are part of the brain's associative networks, the spider-like structures residing in long term memory (Higgins, 1986) that consist of affective and cognitive nodes linked through associative pathways (Anderson, 1983; Fazio, 1986). These nodes contain affective, cognitive, and behavioral components.

Affective forecasting, otherwise known as intuition or the prediction of emotion, also impacts attitude change. Research suggests that predicting emotions is an important component of decision making, in addition to the cognitive processes (Loewenstein, 2007). How we feel about an outcome may override purely cognitive rationales.

Implicit and explicit attitudes

There is also considerable research on *implicit attitudes*, which are generally unacknowledged or outside of awareness, but have effects that are measurable through sophisticated methods using people's response times to stimuli. Implicit and explicit attitudes seem to affect people's behavior, though in different ways. They tend not to be strongly associated with each other, although in some cases they are. The relationship between them is poorly understood.

Why develop a positive attitude?

There is an awakening in the Research and Development organizations and HRD world of the importance of a positive mental attitude. Customers are lost, friction and conflicts occur, stress increases, employees report sick, performance at work gets affected, productivity goes down – all due to a negative mental attitude.

Recent studies in behavioral science and neuroscience reveal scientific proof and evidence of the power of a positive mental attitude. Research also tells us that high achievers have trained themselves in this vital attitude.

HRD in Research and Development organizations must concentrate on cultivate the power of a positive attitude by dealing about the following:

- The core mental states necessary for a positive attitude.
- Overcoming Self limiting thinking.
- Controlling negative thinking and emotions
- Characteristics of negative self-talk.
- Developing the Competency of Optimism.
- How optimists and pessimists respond to failure.
- How to develop a positive attitude.
- Building Self Confidence for a positive attitude.
- Raising Self Image and enhancing Self Esteem.
- Impact of a positive attitude on Body Language, Communication and Relationships.

- How a positive attitude affects performance at work.
- Brain research and the positive attitude.
- The connection between a negative mental attitude and stress.
- Developing Happiness in life

Employees have the ability to transform their life and soar to new heights of success and fulfillment. Whether their attitude is negative... positive... or somewhere in between, HRDs should show them how to take control of their life and unleash their incredible potential by developing positive attitude towards their work, their organization and towards life as a whole.

Communication is the process whereby information is imparted by a sender to a receiver via a *medium*. Communication requires that all parties have an area of communicative commonality. There are *auditory* means, such as speaking, singing and sometimes tone of voice, and *nonverbal*, physical means, such as *body language*, *sign language*, *paralanguage*, *touch*, *eye contact*, by using *writing*. Communication is defined as a process by which we assign and *convey* meaning in an attempt to create shared understanding. This process requires a vast repertoire of skills in *intrapersonal* and *interpersonal* processing, listening, observing, speaking, questioning, analyzing, and evaluating, if you use these processes it is developmental and transfers to all areas of life: home, school, community, work, and beyond. It is through communication that *collaboration* and *cooperation* occur.

Communication is the articulation of sending a message through different media, whether it be verbal or nonverbal, so long as a being transmits a thought provoking idea, *gesture*, action, etc. Communication is a learned skill. Most *babies* are born with the physical ability to make sounds, but must learn to *speak* and communicate effectively. Speaking, *listening*, and our ability to understand verbal and nonverbal meanings are skills we develop in various ways. We learn basic communication skills by observing other people and modeling our behaviors based on what we see. We also are taught some communication skills directly through education, and by practicing those skills and having them evaluated.

Nonetheless, communication is usually described along a few major dimensions: Content (what type of things are communicated), source, emisor, sender or *encoder* (by whom), form (in which form), channel (through which medium), destination, receiver, target or *decoder* (to whom), and the purpose or pragmatic aspect. Between parties, communication includes acts that confer knowledge and experiences, give advice and commands, and ask questions. These acts may take many forms, in one of the various manners of communication. The form depends on the abilities of the group communicating. Together, communication content and form make *messages* that are sent towards a *destination*. The target can be oneself, another *person* or being, another entity (such as a corporation or group of beings).

Communication can be seen as processes of *information transmission* governed by three levels of *semiotic* rules:

1. Syntactic (formal properties of signs and symbols),
2. pragmatic (concerned with the relations between signs/ expressions and their users) and
3. semantic (study of relationships between signs and symbols and what they represent).

Therefore, communication is social interaction where at least two interacting agents share a common set of signs and a common set of *semiotic* rules. This commonly held rule in some sense ignores *autocommunication*, including *intrapersonal communication* via *diaries* or self-talk.

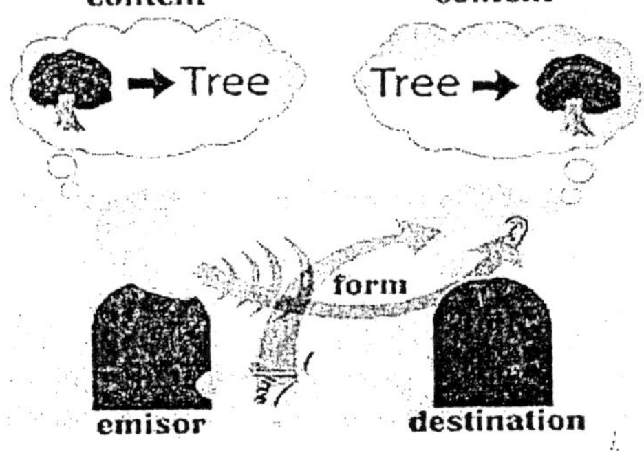

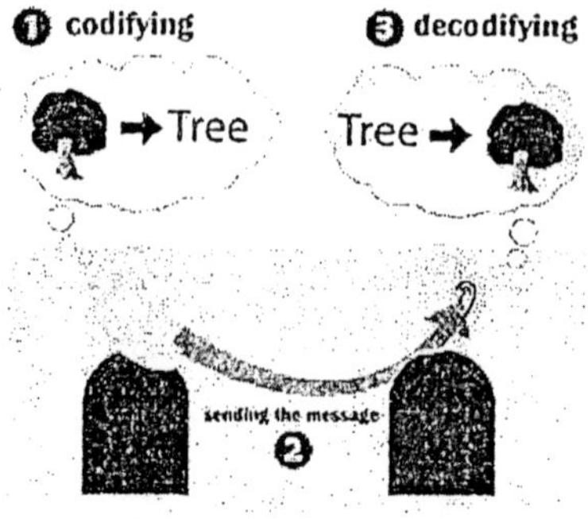

Fig. 7.1: Process of Communication

In a simple model, information or content (e.g. a message in natural language) is sent in some form (as spoken language) from an emisor/ sender/ *encoder* to a destination/ receiver/ *decoder*. In a slightly more complex form a sender and a receiver are linked *reciprocally*. A particular instance of communication is called a *speech act*. In the presence of "*communication noise*" on the transmission channel (air, in this case), reception and decoding of content may be faulty, and thus the speech act may not achieve the desired effect. One problem with this encode-transmit-receive-decode model is that the processes of encoding and decoding imply that the sender and receiver each possess something that functions as a code book, and that these two code books are, at the very least, similar if not identical. Although something like code books is implied by the model, they are nowhere represented in the model, which creates many conceptual difficulties.

Communication happens at many levels (even for one single action), in many different ways, and for most beings, as well as certain machines. Several, if not all, fields of study dedicate a portion of attention to communication, so when speaking about communication it is very important to be sure about what aspects of communication one is speaking about.

Theories of *coregulation* describe communication as a creative and dynamic continuous process, rather than a discrete exchange of information. Canadian media scholar Harold Innis had the theory that people use different types of media to communicate and which one they choose to use will offer different possibilities for the shape and durability of society (Wark, McKenzie 1997). His famous example of this is using ancient Egypt and looking at the ways they built themselves out of media with very different properties stone and papyrus. Papyrus is what he called **'Space Binding'**. It made possible the transmission of written orders across space, empires and enables the waging of distant military campaigns and colonial administration. The other is stone and **'Time Binding'**, through the construction of temples and the pyramids can sustain their authority generation to generation, through this media they can change and shape communication in their society (Wark, McKenzie 1997).

Types of communication

There are 3 major parts in any communication which are body language, voice tonality, and words. According to the research (Mehrabian and Ferris, 'Inference of Attitude from Nonverbal Communication in Two Channels' in *The Journal of Counselling Psychology* Vol. 31, 1967, pp. 248-52), 55% of impact is determined by body language—postures, gestures, and eye contact, 38% by the tone of voice, and 7% by the content or the words used in the communication process. Although the exact percentage of influence may differ from variables such as the listener and the speaker, communication as a whole strives for the same goal and thus, in some cases, can be universal. System of signals, such as voice sounds, intonations or pitch, gestures or *written* symbols which communicate thoughts or feelings. If a language is about communicating with signals, voice, sounds, gestures, or written symbols, can animal communications be considered as a language? Animals do not have a written form of a language, but use a language to communicate with each another. In that sense, an animal communication can be considered as a separate language.

Human spoken and written languages can be described as a *system* of *symbols* (sometimes known as *lexemes*) and the *grammars* (*rules*) by which the symbols are manipulated. The word "language" is also used to refer to common properties of languages. Language learning is normal in human childhood. Most human languages use patterns of *sound* or *gesture* for symbols which enable communication with others around them. There are thousands of human languages, and these seem to share certain properties, even though many shared properties have exceptions.

Dialogue

A dialogue is a *reciprocal conversation* between two or more entities. The *etymological* origins of the word (in *Greek* äéÜ(diá, through) + ëüãïò (logos, word, speech) concepts like flowing-through meaning) do not necessarily convey the way in which people have come to use the word, with some confusion between the prefix äéÜ- (diá-,through) and the prefix äé- (di-, two) leading to the assumption that a dialogue is necessarily between only two parties.

Non verbal communication

Nonverbal communication is the process of communicating through sending and receiving wordless *messages*. Such messages can be communicated through *gesture*, *body language* or *posture*; *facial expression* and eye contact, object communication such as *clothing*, *hairstyles* or even *architecture*, or symbols and *infographics*, as well as through an aggregate of the above, such as *behavioral communication*. Speech may also contain nonverbal elements known as *paralanguage*, including voice quality, emotion and speaking style, as well as prosodic features such as *rhythm*, *intonation* and *stress*. Likewise, written texts have nonverbal elements such as handwriting style, spatial arrangement of words, or the use of *emoticons*. A portmanteau of the English words emotion (or emote) and icon, an emoticon is a symbol or combination of symbols used to convey emotional content in written or message form.

Communications theorist *James W. Carey* draws on the notion that "society exists not only by transmission, by communication, but [also] in transmission, in communication", claiming that "societies distribute information...and that by such transactions and the channels of communication peculiar to them society is made possible"

From this, he suggests two ways of viewing the communication process and the relationship between transmitter and receiver which demonstrate differing ideas of how communication and society are integrated. These are as follows:

- *Transmission model*: communication as simply a process whereby messages are transmitted and distributed in space for the control of distance and people. A somewhat hierarchical view, where the communicating or gaining of knowledge is of the most importance.
- *Ritual model*: the maintenance of society in time through the representation of shared beliefs. Invites participation on the basis of our assuming, where communication produces social bonds which tie men and women together and make associated life possible by way of shared information.

In order for a Research and Development organization to be successful in the global context, its personnel should be aware and conscious of communication protocols.

TEAM BUILDING

Team building is another approach that would add strength to Research and Development. After all, it is not individuals who embark on the innovation journey, but a number of teams working together. The term team building generally refers to the selection, development, and collective motivation of result-oriented *teams*. Team Building is the process of improving collective performance.

Cummings and Worley (2001) define team building as "the process of helping a work group become more effective in accomplishing its tasks and satisfying the needs of group members" (p. 676).

Team Vs Group

A team differs from a group. A group is a set of people with individual objectives who happen to share the same boss, or the same workplace, or be part of the same organizational unit. In a group, individuals might even have the same objectives - e.g.: in a sales force, everyone might have the same sales target to meet, but they may also compete against each other rather than cooperate.

A team is a group that works towards a single, common objective. In fact, they might have different individual objectives, but those objectives contribute to the higher collective one. E.g. in a sales team, one person might make appointments, another provide technical sales support, another prepare a bid document, and another make the sale. But they are all accountable together for the sales and are not judged solely on individual objectives.

When a *team* in an *organizational development* context embarks upon a *process* of *self-assessment* in order to gauge its own effectiveness and thereby improve performance, it can be argued that it is engaging in team building. The great success of the Japanese has beet attributed to their instined Team work. Team work in simple terms is "the ability of a group of people to cooperate and work effectively together, the possibility of each participant to think and act for the group rather than for his own personal benefit"

The process of team building includes,

- clarifying the goal, and building ownership across the team
- identifying the inhibitors to teamwork and removing or overcoming them, or if they cannot be removed, mitigating their negative effect on the team.

Steps of Team Building

Team building is pursued via a variety of practices, such as group self-assessment and *group-dynamic games*, and generally sits within the theory and practice of *organizational development.*

There are 10 steps of Team building and they are given as below:

1. Getting Upper-Management Support
2. Define the purpose of team
3. Identify Time Frames
4. Select Team members
5. Team-Member openings
6. Share the overall purpose
7. Team Name
8. Create the team mission statement and goals
9. Core Team Issues
10. Establishing team norms

A simple but effective methodology involves:

- Establishing **ownership** of shared goals
- **Removing inhibitors/blockages** to achievement of those goals
- **Introducing enablers** (awareness, resources, information, processes, etc.) to help achieve those goals
- Using team building processes (e.g.: health checks, performance management, 360 feedback) in **the correct sequence** to gradually raise performance, akin to climbing a ladder one rung at a time

Team Building is often ineffective because:

- In many cases, advanced techniques are used whilst there is a lack of buy in to the shared objectives

  (commitment to team building activities is predicated on commitment to the overall direction/goals)
- Interventions are made out of sequence

  (e.g.: a poorly defined structure, roles and responsibilities will undermine attempts to improve interpersonal relationships)
- Many offsite events fail to add any real, lasting value because the approach taken to team building is too generic

  (any offsite event should be designed to meet specific goals and outcomes)
- There is often a lack of understanding of the difference between a group and a team

Team building with a group can be counter-productive, detracting from individual performance without any compensatory collective benefit.

- There is a lack of assessment of the team

  (diagnosis is required in order to develop effective intervention strategies)

Team Building Stages:

- Forming,

- Storming,
- Norming,
- Performing

In the Forming stage (*Forming-Storming-Norming-Performing*), individuals are committed, at most, to their own objectives. Members will only invest time in Storming activities if they think it is worth it - that is, if the collective objectives are seen as important as their own.

A common mistake is for individuals to think that being committed to their own objectives means they are committed to the team. As in the age-old metaphor where a house needs to be built on rock, the foundation of all team building is commitment to the shared goal.

Techniques of Team Building

If team building is viewed as a commodity, as a product to be purchased from a supplier, then it is unlikely to have any lasting value. Having an awayday, playing games or doing fun things will generally lead to lasting and improved collective performance only in the context of a good plan, where events are bespoke (designed to meet specific objectives and outcomes). In fact, having an awayday without good design is taking a gamble - it may achieve something, be a waste of time, or even damage teamwork.

The choice of intervention strategy depends not only on the current state of teamwork, but on the nature of the people. For highly motivated individuals, it can be enough to set a high level direction and then allow individuals to contribute to the detailed development of the goals. For others, whose natural motivations are more individual, there may need to be objective-based rewards that require teamwork. In some instances, where high levels of teamwork cannot be achieved, they may only be effective in the Forming stage, which is highly dependent on leadership.

Strategies

Interventions fall into four main areas:

- **Individual** - e.g.: development of individual skills; establishing familiarity with shared processes

- **Relational** - e.g.: improvement of unconscious dynamics; engendering a sense of common purpose and commitment
- **In/Out Groups** - tackling the barriers between different organizational units
- **Cultural** - building a teamwork ethos in larger organizations

  To assess itself, a team seeks *feedback* to find out both:

  - its current strengths as a team and
  - its current weakness

To improve its current performance, a team uses the feedback from the team assessment in order to:

- identify any gap between the desired state and the actual state
- design a gap-closure strategy

Team building is pursued via a variety of practices, such as group self-assessment and *group-dynamic games*, and generally sits within the theory and practice of *organizational development*.

Although, individual ability and motivation are important, efficiency as a group is treated as multiplier factor for productivity. Indeed team work at all levels is highly valued and carefully nurtured. Team spirit is to be inculcated amongst the employees of Research and development organizations. Individuals possessing team building capacities are needed in any Research and Development organization for their development since the activities in these organizations need individuals to works in teams.

Successful team building will have far reaching ramifications in a research and development organization. It brings about improvement in the way team members interact and in their ability to solve problems. Better problem–solving means better efficiency in general. Increased efficiency tends to boost morale and productivity. It also helps to decrease stress, turnover and operating costs. And all of these improvements bolster the organizations public image. Once established an effective team becomes self perpetuating.

LEADERSHIP

Discussions about leadership today have become so frequent and impassioned, that they have become almost evangelical in tone.

Leading is a very human activity — everyone's human — so every human can be trained for good leadership. We associate any desirable trait to what leaders should be. People exhort others to become better leaders, to more effectively manage change, etc. Students find it fascinating to read about leadership, to research aspects of leadership, etc. Current publications about research and development organizations often have the term "leadership" in the title.

While this trend shows us the critical importance of leadership and sometimes has greatly inspired us on to greater achievements in life and work, it has also helped people to become more effective in organizations.

Many people today are seeking to understand — and many people are writing about — the concept and practices of leadership. There are a great many reasons for the popularity of the concept, including that organizations are faced with changes like never before. The concept of leadership is relevant to any aspect of ensuring effectiveness in organizations and in managing change.

There has been an explosion of literature about leadership lately. Leadership is an important dimension that can be used to get the best from a research and development organization. An origination having good leadership provides a base for its productivity improvement. A good leader having key leadership skills can make a difference in any research and development organization. This can make a difference at the operational level by reducing the time it takes to do things. Any research and development organization without effective leadership has to work harder and harder to get the work done and is also prone to more and more mistakes.

Leadership is one of the most salient aspects of the organizational context. However, defining leadership has been challenging. The following sections discuss several important aspects of leadership including a description of what leadership is and a description of several popular theories and styles of leadership. It also dives into topics such as the role of emotions and vision, as well as leadership effectiveness and performance.

What is Leadership?

Leading is a very human activity. Many people believe that leadership is simply being the first, biggest or most powerful. Leadership in organizations has a different and more meaningful definition.

Very simply put, a leader is interpreted as someone who sets direction in an effort and influences people to follow that direction. How they set that direction and influence people depends on a variety of factors that we'll consider.

Oxford English Dictionary traces the word "leadership" in English only as far back as the 19th century.

Leadership has been described as the *"process of social influence in which one person is able to enlist the aid and support of others in the accomplishment of a common task".*

A definition which is more inclusive is given by Alan Keith of Genentech who said

"Leadership is ultimately about creating a way for people to contribute to making something extraordinary happen."

Leadership Cube

Different people tend to talk about leadership from many different perspectives and not even realize that they are doing so. It is very simplistic to generalize about leadership as if the term applies the same way in every situation. To really understand leadership, one must understand "Leadership Cube." The Cube represents at least 20 different perspectives on leadership.

The Cube includes the following dimensions:

1. five domains of leadership
2. two contexts of leadership
3. two orientations of leadership

Imagine each of these 3 dimensions along one side of a box, or cube. That would produce a cube with 20 smaller cells (5 times 2 times 2 = 20). Each of the 20 cells represents a unique perspective on leadership, Research, discussions, etc.

Five Domains of Leadership

Domain	Relevant Leadership Skills
Leading yourself	Time management, stress management, assertiveness, etc.
Leading other individuals	Coaching, mentoring, delegating, etc.
Leading other groups	Meeting management, facilitation skills, etc.
Leading organizations	Strategic planning, Balanced Scorecard, etc.

Two Contexts of Leadership

Context	Focus of Context
Roles	Board Chair, Chief Executive Officer, executive roles, etc.

Two Orientations of Leadership

Orientation	Leadership Values
Results-oriented	Timeliness, efficiency, work direction, authority, etc.
Relationship-oriented	Participation, empowerment, relationships, etc.

To really comprehend the "territory" of leadership, you should briefly scan some of the major theories, notice various styles of leadership and review some of the suggested traits and characteristics that leaders should have.

Leadership Styles

Leaders carry out their roles in a wide variety of styles, e.g., autocratic, democratic, participatory, laissez-faire (hands off), etc. Often, the leadership style depends on the situation, including the life cycle of the organization. *Sanskrit* literature identifies ten types of leaders.

How Do Leaders Lead?

The particular competencies (knowledge, skills and abilities) that a person needs in order to lead at a particular time in an organization depend on a variety of factors, including:

1. Whether that person is leading one other individual, a group or a large organization;
2. The extent of leadership skills that person already has;
3. That person's basic nature and values (competencies should be chosen that are in accordance with that nature and those values);
4. Whether the group or organization is for-profit or nonprofit, new or long-established, and large or small;
5. The particular culture (or values and associated behaviors) of whomever is being led.

MOTIVATION

In today's knowledge-centric era, employees of an organization have emerged as one of the most important elements determining long-term success of organizations. There are many dimensions to optimizing the organizational environment in order to improve productivity through improved employee motivation. Organizations are, increasingly, devising systems and tools for motivating employees and encouraging them to bring out the 'best' in them at the workplace. Performance-based-pay is one such tool.

Motivation is the set of reasons that determines one to engage in a particular behavior. The term is generally used for human motivation but, theoretically, it can be used to describe the causes for animal behavior as well. In research and development organisation we refer to human motivation.

According to various theories, motivation may be rooted in the basic need to minimize physical pain and maximize pleasure, or it may include specific needs such as eating and resting, or a desired object, hobby, *goal*, state of being, *ideal*, or it may be attributed to less-apparent reasons such as *altruism*, *morality*, or avoiding *mortality*.

A *reward*, tangible or intangible, is presented after the occurrence of an action (i.e. behavior) with the intent to cause the behavior to occur again. This is done by *associating* positive meaning to the behavior. Studies show that if the person receives the reward immediately, the effect would be greater, and decreases as duration lengthens. Repetitive action-reward combination can cause the action to become *habit*. Motivation comes from two things: you, and other people. There is extrinsic motivation, which comes from others, and intrinsic motivation, which comes from within you.

Some authors distinguish between two forms of intrinsic motivation: one based on *enjoyment*, the other on obligation. In this context, *obligation* refers to motivation based on what an individual thinks ought to be done. For instance, a feeling of responsibility for a mission may lead to helping others beyond what is easily observable, rewarded, or fun.

A *reinforcer* is different from reward, in that reinforcement is intended to create a measured increase in the rate of a desirable behavior following the addition of something to the environment.

Intrinsic and extrinsic motivation

Intrinsic motivation

Intrinsic motivation occurs when people engage in an activity, such as a *hobby*, without obvious external incentives. This form of motivation has been studied by *social* and *educational* psychologists since the early 1970s. Research has found that it is usually associated with high educational achievement and enjoyment by students. Intrinsic motivation has been explained by Fritz Heider's *attribution theory*, Bandura's work on *self-efficacy*, and Ryan and Deci's cognitive evaluation theory. Employees or students are likely to be intrinsically motivated if they:

- attribute their work/ educational results to internal factors that they can control (e.g. the amount of effort they put in),
- believe they can be effective agents in reaching desired goals (i.e. the results are not determined by luck),
- are interested in mastering a topic, rather than just rote-learning to achieve good grades.

In knowledge-sharing communities and organizations, people often cite altruistic reasons for their participation, including contributing to a common good, a moral obligation to the group, mentorship or 'giving back'. In *work* environments, *money* may provide a more powerful extrinsic factor than the intrinsic motivation provided by an enjoyable workplace.

In terms of sports, intrinsic motivation is the motivation that comes from inside the performer. That is, the athlete competes for the love of the sport.

Extrinsic motivation

Extrinsic motivation comes from outside of the performer. Money is the most obvious example, but *coercion* and threat of punishment are also common extrinsic motivations.

In sports, the crowd may cheer the performer on, and this motivates him or her to do well. Trophies are also extrinsic incentives. Competition is often extrinsic because it encourages the performer to win and beat others, not to enjoy the intrinsic rewards of the activity.

Social psychological research has indicated that extrinsic rewards can lead to *overjustification* and a subsequent reduction in intrinsic motivation.

Self-control in Motivation

Self-control of motivation is increasingly understood as a subset of *emotional intelligence*; a person may be highly intelligent according to a more conservative definition (as measured by many *intelligence tests*), yet unmotivated to dedicate this intelligence to certain tasks. *Yale School of Management* professor *Victor Vroom*'s "*expectancy theory*" provides an account of when people will decide whether to exert self control to pursue a particular goal.

Drives and desires can be described as *a deficiency or need that activates behaviour that is aimed at a goal or an incentive.* These are thought to originate within the individual and may not require external stimuli to encourage the behaviour. Basic drives could be sparked by deficiencies such as hunger, which motivates a person to seek food; whereas more subtle drives might be the desire for praise and approval, which motivates a person to behave in a manner pleasing to others.

By contrast, the role of extrinsic rewards and stimuli can be seen in the example of training animals by giving them treats when they perform a trick correctly. The treat motivates the animals to perform the trick consistently, even later when the treat is removed from the process.

ACTION RESEARCH IN HRD

Action Research is a structured approach to inquiry: Problem Formation, Data Collection, Data Analysis, Reporting Results and Action Planning,

Action Research is disciplined inquiry by practitioners working to investigate issues related to performance improvement. They assume responsibility for developing their own knowledge and understanding, thus enhancing their profession practice.

Action research is focused on immediate application, not on the development of theory or on generalization of applications. It places emphasis on problem faced and in local setting. Its findings are to be evaluated in terms of local applicability, and not on universal validity. Its purpose is to improve HRD practices and at the same time improve the personnel who try to improve the HRD practices: to combine the research processes, habits of thinking, ability to work harmoniously with others, and professional spirit.

If most HRD personnel are to be involved in research activity, it will probably be in the area of action research. Modest studies may be conducted for the purpose of trying to improve local HRD practices in their organization. Though fundamental research must continue to make its essential contribution to behavioral theory and applied research to the improvement of HRD practices, these activities will be primarily the function of professional researchers, many of them subsidized by universities, private and government agencies, professional associations, and philanthropic foundations.

Action research applies scientific thinking and methods to real-life problems and represents a great improvement over manager's subjective judgments and decisions based on personal experience. Action research in HR practices and activities gives the extent of success or failures of policies and practices. It provides an understanding of practices, policies that are successful and those which are not, what changes are necessary and in what area of personnel management.

Personnel research is the "task of searching for and analyzing facts, to understand how personnel problems may be solved or principles governing their solutions derived. It implies searching investigations, re-examinations, re-assessment and reevaluations. It is purposive and systematic investigation designed to test considered hypothesis or thorough framed questions.

The continuous change in technology, business management and, innovations in psychology, sociology make it necessary for the Human Resources Specialist to search new methods, practices that keeps pace with challenging needs for growth and improving the existing practices. It aims at examining and evaluating the existing practices, programmes, policies and modify these due to changed circumstances and work environments.

Characteristic of Action Research in HRD

- It is purposive. It seeks answers to questions.
- It is spiral.
- It is objective- recognizes and limits bias and prejudice in every step of the process
- It is systematic involving a comprehensive design. Investigations are conducted on a design or plan.
- It is planned and designed investigation analysis and helps in fact finding
- It aims at improving present practices in HRD or at finding solutions to problems faced in HRD

Objectives of Action Research in HRD

The primary objective is evaluative, to evaluate the present HRD practices and policies. It aims at:

- Evaluating present practices, conditions and activities.
- To appraise, proposals in respect of HR policies and activities

- To find and propose ways and means of strengthening the abilities and attitudes of employees at high level on a continuing basis by new techniques.
- To evaluate and review linkages between organizational strategies and HRD strategies
- To modify, amend existing HR practices as per need or replace with new practices

Steps of Action Research

- Problem formulation
- Selection of probable causes: framing hypotheses
- Designing procedures to test the hypotheses
- Choice of methodology
- Data collection-through various tools and techniques
- Analysis of data
- Interpretation, finding and conclusion.

A few problems on which action research in HRD could be carried out are as follows:

- To find the effectiveness of HRM on the strategic management decisions to achieve overall objectives and goals of the organization
- To find the effect of training and development on the performance of human resources and its contribution in success and growth of an organization
- Study the effect of styles of leadership on the management and find out the effect of different styles of leadership on the stability and growth of the organization
- Study the effect of compensation including incentives, rewards and other monetary benefits, on the performance and contribution by human resource towards achieving goals of the organization
- Study various motivational techniques used by organization and its effect on the performance of human resources and understand what contribution is made and the role played by human resources towards the success of the organization.

- Action research on each major function performed by HRD can be undertaken to make inquiries, investigations, which will be useful and help in improving the role of HRD.

Wendell L French and Cecil Bell define **organization development** (OD) at one point as "organization improvement through action research". If one idea can be said to summarize OD's underlying philosophy, it would be action research as it was conceptualized by *Kurt Lewin* and later elaborated and expanded on by other behavioral scientists. Concerned with social change and, more particularly, with effective, permanent social change, Lewin believed that the motivation to change was strongly related to action: If people are active in decisions affecting them, they are more likely to adopt new ways. "Rational social management", he said, "proceeds in a spiral of steps, each of which is composed of a circle of planning, action, and fact-finding about the result of action".

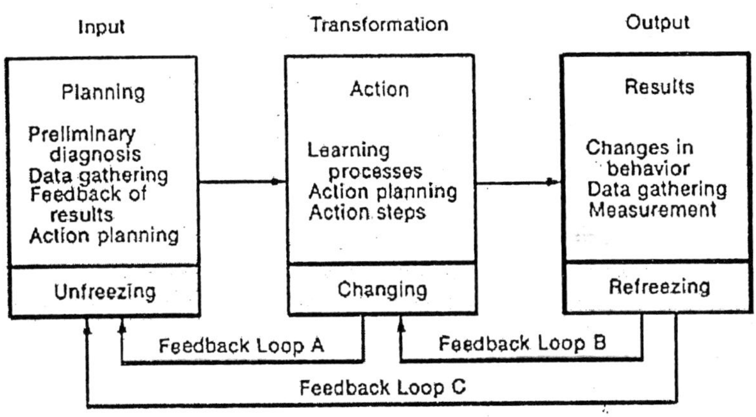

Fig. 7.2: Systems Model of Action-Research Process

Lewin's description of the process of change involves three steps:

Unfreezing: Faced with a dilemma or disconfirmation, the individual or group becomes aware of a need to change.

Changing: The situation is diagnosed and new models of behavior are explored and tested.

Refreezing: Application of new behavior is evaluated, and if reinforcing, adopted.

Figure 7.2 summarizes the steps and processes involved in planned change through action research. Action research is depicted as a cyclical process of change. **The cycle begins** with a series of planning actions initiated by the client and the change agent working together. The principal elements of this stage include a preliminary diagnosis, data gathering, feedback of results, and joint action planning. In the language of systems theory, this is the input phase, in which the client system becomes aware of problems as yet unidentified, realizes it may need outside help to effect changes, and shares with the consultant the process of problem diagnosis.

The second stage of action research is the action, or transformation, phase. This stage includes actions relating to learning processes (perhaps in the form of role analysis) and to planning and executing behavioral changes in the client organization. As shown in Figure 1, feedback at this stage would move via Feedback Loop A and would have the effect of altering previous planning to bring the learning activities of the client system into better alignment with change objectives. Included in this stage is action-planning activity carried out jointly by the consultant and members of the client system. Following the workshop or learning sessions, these action steps are carried out on the job as part of the transformation stage.

The third stage of action research is the output, or results, phase. This stage includes actual changes in behavior (if any) resulting from corrective action steps taken following the second stage. Data are again gathered from the client system so that progress can be determined and necessary adjustments in learning activities can be made. Minor adjustments of this nature can be made in learning activities via Feedback Loop B (see *Fig. 7.1*). Major adjustments and reevaluations would return the OD project to the first, or planning, stage for basic changes in the program. The action-research model shown in *Figure 1* closely follows Lewin's repetitive cycle of planning, action, and measuring results. It also illustrates other aspects of Lewin's general model of change. As indicated in the diagram, the planning stage is a period of unfreezing, or problem awareness. The action stage is a period of changing, that is, trying out new forms of behavior in an effort to understand and cope with the system's problems. (There is inevitable overlap between the stages, since the boundaries are not clear-cut and cannot be in a continuous process). The results stage is a period of refreezing, in which new behaviors are tried out on the job and, if successful and reinforcing, become a part of the system's repertoire of problem-solving behavior.

Action research is problem centered, client centered, and action oriented. It involves the system in a diagnostic, active-learning, problem-finding, and problem-solving process. Data are not simply returned in the form of a written report but instead are fed back in open joint sessions, and the client and the change agent collaborate in identifying and ranking specific problems, in devising methods for finding their real causes, and in developing plans for coping with them realistically and practically. Scientific method in the form of data gathering, forming hypotheses, testing hypotheses, and measuring results, although not pursued as rigorously as in the laboratory, is nevertheless an integral part of the process. Action research also sets in motion a long-range, cyclical, self-correcting mechanism for maintaining and enhancing the effectiveness of the system by leaving the system with practical and useful tools for self-analysis and self-renewal.

HRD APPROACHES

As you already know, HRD is the process of increasing the knowledge, the skills, and the capacities of all the people in the society. In economic terms, it could be described as the accumulation of human capital and its effective investment ion the development of an economy. In political terms, HRD prepares people of adult participation in political process, particularly as citizens in a democracy. From the social and cultural point of view, the development to human resources help people to lead fuller and richer lives, less bound by tradition. In short, the process of human resource development unlocks the door for a better and fuller life in a society.

There were three distinct approaches to HRD in 1960's and 1970's. They were:

1. Human Capital Approach
2. Social Psychological Approach
3. Poverty Alleviation Approach

These approaches are represented by Schultz from the economics tradition, McClelland from the Social psychology base and the World Bank in Poverty Alleviation point of view. There are a few similarities in these three approaches. All these three approaches stress on human competency development and role of education in developing human competencies.

Human Capital Approach is based on human capital as a human resource. In economic terms human resource development was equated with human capital formation in the early years. Human capital consist of various activities and Schultz analyzed five areas namely, health, on-the-job training, formal education, adult literacy programmes, nutritional status.

People acquire useful skills and knowledge but they are not a form of capital, it is a substantial part of a product of deliberate investment. Increases in the national output have been largely compared with increase of land, man-hours and physical reproducible capital.

Scultz presented several inferences supporting the linkage between economic growth and human capital. He argued that large differences in earnings between whites and blacks working on comparable activities, between those in south and north etc. are reflections of differences in education and health. For example: Most migratory farm workers earn very little as compared to others and they have virtually no schooling, are poor in health, unskilled and have little ability to do useful work. By this he brought out the importance of investing in human capital. The poor countries which get capital from outside invest for the formation of structural equipment and some times also into inventories. But it is generally not available for additional investments in man. Consequently human capabilities do not stay abreast of physical capital and they do become limiting factors in economic growth. According to Scultz the most distinctive feature of our economic system is the growth in human capital.

Without it there would be only hard manual work and poverty except for those who have income form poverty.

Social Psychological Approach highlights that motivation, attitudes and values are important variables in development. In the early 20th century, McClelland examined the factors contributing to the economic development of various countries. He examined achievement motivation of people. The achievement motivation is the concern of the people to achieve same thing of excellence unique or something different than anything before and to do better than before. For this purpose he analysed children's stories and other popular literature of those countries and came to know that those countries, which have advanced economically, showed evidence of achievement motivation. His analysis suggested the evidence of achievement motivation. It suggested that the way children are socialized, the nature of socialization process, etc., determined whether they would undertake entrepreneurial activities and contribute to economic development. His analysis suggests that the degree of challenges offered by the environment, child-rearing practices in the family, interaction pattern of parents with their children, interactive factors associated with religion and social class and core religions and social values, all influence achievement motivation, which in-turn influence economic development.

Thus McClelland, after analyzing a number of studies, Psychological, Sociological, anthropological and other social sciences, recommended that those countries, which are involved in economic development should pay proper attention to the inculcation of values in children to create achievement motivation later in their lives. Scultz goes a little further and suggests the ways and means of developing achievement motivation among its people.

Thus we see that entrepreneurial spirit can be developed through achievement motivation and training given to the youths and adults. This is seen to be successful in many countries including India.

Poverty Alleviation approach is a recent approach towards HRD. Alleviation of poverty is the way. A key focus was given by World Development report 1990, in which the poverty alleviation programmes are acknowledged as one of the effective ways of investing in human beings. This report has also identified the existing problem and argued that investments in human development are necessary to help poor to help themselves. The ways suggested for human development through poverty alleviation are getting rid of hunger, limiting family size, providing at least primary education and such other programmes which are generally welcomed accepted universally. While recognizing the importance of human capital formation through education, health and such other programmes, it suggests that state interventions are needed to develop and alleviate or reduce poverty.

Systems Approach: Systems approach can institutionalize HRD and facilitate its contributions.

There are various systems of HRD

1. Career System
   a. Manpower planning Recruitment development
   b. Potential appraisals and research promotions
   c. Career planning and development
2. Work planning
   a. Role analysis (goal setting)
   b. Contextual analysis
   c. Performance appraisal
3. Development system
   a. Training and learning
   b. Performance coaching / counseling
   c. Others like Job rotation, mentoring
   d. Staff (worker) development
4. Self Renewal system
   a. Role efficacy
   b. Organization
   c. Action oriented
5. Culture System
   a. HRD climate

b. Values
c. Quality orientation
d. Reward and recognition
e. Information
f. Communication
g. Empowerment

The modern approaches to HRD in any organization include:

1. Top-down to Bottom-up Approach
2. Micro to Macro Approach
3. Generic to Specific Approach
4. Open to Closed Approach

These HRD approaches assume that employees engage in learning to acquire skills and knowledge which help in organizational development.

The *Top-down to Bottom-up approach* emphasises on giving priority for greater awareness building of the general mass rather than to provide highly technical expertise to the handful of professionals. It emphsises on imparting training from the top executive level rather than from the operational level.

In the *Micro to Macro approach* emphasis is on practical training in micro level to the public and local bodies rather than highly advanced courses and training in macro level.

The *Generic to Specific approach* makes a broad distinction between generic knowledge or skills and domain specific knowledge or skills. Generic knowledge and skills can be used in a variety of situation. The ability or manipulate things with our fingers is a generic skill with applications in feeding, dressing, turning pages. Domain specific knowledge and skills relate to particular area or domains of our experience. The ability to drive a car is a skill specific to road transport. Knowledge of attributes of an atom is domain specific and is unlikely to be used outside specialized fields or particle physics.

Someone who is already knolwledgeable or skillful in a specific domain finds it easier to assimilate further knowledge or skill within the same domain because there is already a framework to which to relate the new information. With generic sills and knowledge, we find that we learn them once then apply them again and again. We may, however, be able to refine our knowledge and skills be reflection on our use of them. The Generic to Specific approach prioritizes generic type of training and courses rather than specific highly sophisticated program of HRD.

The *Open to Closed approach* of HRD emphsises on facilitating training and other learning opportunities open to all rather than limiting to the certain groups on a closed basis.

SUMMARY

Action Research is disciplined inquiry by practitioners working to investigate issues related to performance improvement. They assume responsibility for developing their own knowledge and understanding, thus enhancing their profession practice. Action research is depicted as a cyclical process of change. The cycle begins with a series of planning actions initiated by the client and the change agent working together. The principal elements of this stage include a preliminary diagnosis, data gathering, feedback of results, and joint action planning.

As HRD came to prominence many models came into existence. Some of these are: The strategic HR framework, The activities for management of Firm infrastructure, The Integrative framework, Human Capital Appraisal Approach, HRD Score Card Approach and the P-CMM Approach.

UNIT 8

PROFESSIONALIZATION IN HUMAN RESOURCE DEVELOPMENT

INTRODUCTION

It is more than three decades since the term Human Resource Development became popular in the country. In 1975, a dedicated department to promote Human Resources Development was initiated in India at Larsen and Toubro Limited. Since then, by the mid 80's a large number of organizations in India had established HRD departments. By the mid 80's, HR had become an accepted role and most organizations had changed their personnel, training and other related functions to HRD. Since then HRD has come to mean new expectations, a new knowledge and a new function.

Concerns about professionalism and professionalization of HRD have been in existence since the last decade. The issue of professionalizing HRD was taken up by the National HRD Network in their symposium in 1990. Before looking into professionalization of HRD, let us have a look of what is a profession, how it differs form an occupation and the characteristics of a profession.

What is a profession?

According to the Webster Dictionary: 'A profession is an open declaration or avowal of belief or opinion', and professions are distinct form a simple collection of people doing similar work or other non-professional groups by their efforts to define expected norms of ethical behavior among their members. For the members of a profession, 'ethical standards are central to understanding what constitutes proper conduct as well as expectations of virtues professionals should possess' (Gellerman, Frankel, and Kadenson, 1990).

Occupation differs from profession. Occupation is that which occupies or engages the time and attention, the principal business of one's life. An occupation metamorphoses into a profession if it is well practiced and developed by practitioners. To some extent an occupation exhibits the characteristics of professionalization.

The core characteristics of a profession are prolonged specialized training in a body of abstract knowledge and a collective or service orientation. Let us look into the various characteristics of profession given by various thinkers and subsequently analyze the characteristics of HRD as a profession.

Goode (1960) proposes the following characteristics of profession:

- A profession determines its own standards of education
- The student of a profession goes through a more far-reaching adult socialization experience than a learner in another occupation
- Professional practice is often legally recognized by some form of licensure
- Licensing and admission boards are manned by the members of the profession
- Most legislation concerned with the profession is shaped by that profession
- An occupation is known for its gains in income, power and prestige. It can demand high-caliber students
- The practitioner is relatively free of lay evaluation and control
- The norms of practice enforced by the profession are more stringent than legal controls
- Members are more strongly identified and affiliated with the profession, than are members of the occupation
- The profession is more likely to be a terminal occupation. Members do not care to leave it and a higher proportion assert that if they had to do it all over again, they would again choose same type of work.

Barber (1963) lists the characteristics of a profession. They are:

- A high degree of generalized and systematic knowledge
- Primary orientation to the community interest rather than to individual self interest
- A high degree of self control of behaviour through codes of ethics internalized in the process of work socialization and through voluntary associations organized and operated by work specialists themselves
- A system of rewards (monetary and non-monetary), that is primarily a set of symbols of work achievement and thus ends in themselves, not means to some end of individual self-interest.

Harries-Jenkins (1970) identifies the following elements of professionalization.

1. *Structural Element*
    - Specialization: the exclusive nature of group activity
    - Centralization: the locus of authority-sanctions mechanism
    - Standardization: the control of non-occupational behaviour
2. *Contextual Element*
    - Spatio-temporal dimension
    - Size of occupational group
    - Resources of occupational group
    - Group relations
3. *Activity Element*
    - The goals of occupational group
    - The role of individual members
4. *Educational Element*
    - Occupational intelligence requirements
    - Basis of systematic theory
    - Institutionalized educational process
    - Length of training
    - Cost of training
5. *Ideological Element*
    - Personality involvement

- Sense of group identity
- Group culture
- Status
- Socialization process

6. *Behavioural Element*
   - Code of conduct
   - Evaluation of merit

Based on these criteria, HRD can be identified as a profession today. The following analysis of facts regarding HRD is presented to have a view of the professionalization of HRD.

1. Knowledge Base of HRD in India

There is a well developed knowledge base in HRD. The knowledge deals with various aspects of HRD like: concept of HRD, designing HRD systems, organization development and change management, Career planning and development, performance management, feedback and appraisals, counselling, organizational learning, training and development, organizational behavior and personal growth, basic psychology and principles of psychology, creativity, HRD for different categories of people.

It has also derived its knowledge base form other fields like Education, Psychology and Organization Behaviour. The body of knowledge is growing continuously due to contributions by various researches in all areas of HRD.

2. Requirements to be called an HRD professional

The role of an HRD professional is well defined. The Academy of HRD (AHRD) formulated a standard for HRD professionals.

There is a discrepancy in the course content and also the name of the degree offered. Persons with MBA with HRD specialization, or MSW with HRD specialization, diploma in PGDHRD/HRM/PM & IR may acquire a job in HRD. This is not so in other professions like medicine and law. It is also high time that the pre-requisites for this profession are defined, since, any graduate who has studied arts, commerce or science and mathematics or even computers, can take up a course in management. Well defined pre-requisites for a course are essential for practicing a profession.

3. Education and Training facilities for HRD

Recently, a number of institutions have started programs in HRD. While professional bodies like the All India Management Association and Universities like IGNOU offer diploma, certification and masters programs. But it is seen that these courses in various institutions and its curricula are not standardized. There is an urgent need to standardize academic preparation and curricula.

4. Legal recognition and standards of HRD profession-Licensing requirements

The most important aspect of professionalization is the existence of licensing association. Registration of medical practitioners and The Bar Association for Law are a few examples. No person can legally practice these professions without being enrolled in these associations. In the field of HRD, though associations like All India Management Association exists, registration and licensing is not mandatory for practicing the profession. In future if HRD professionalization is required, government bodies recognize a licensing procedure.

5. Services offered by the Profession and their availability

Case studies have shown that certain services like, counseling, OD interventions, facilitation of learning, team building, potential assessment etc., offered by HRD professionals are successful. Services offered by HRD needs to be defined and publicized.

6. Sense of Identity and Belongingness in the profession (HRD Community)

Network and ASTD have facilitated the development of a common identity, but it is not strong. It is high time for these bodies to start a separate professional membership with people possessing the required qualification and through assessment of appropriateness of the member.

7. Code of conduct and Ethics

A code of ethics called the Standards of Ethics was introduced by the members of Academy of Human Resource Development, USA to establish desired standards of behavior and to bring in an increased sense of professionalism to those doing HRD research and practice and to develop integrity. The general principles on which it was based are: competence, integrity, professional responsibility, respect for people's right and dignity, concern for others' welfare, social responsibility.

There is no accepted and enforced code of conduct or ethics for HRD personnel in India. Though the National HRD Network has constituted a committee to formulate standards of conduct, ethics, and values, the committee has not come up with it.

8. Public Acceptance and Well-defined Member Roles

Like in medicine and law, public recognition is a very important aspect of any profession. This is because they deal with issues concerning the public and society and offer their services directly to the public. But for HRD its clients are organizations and their employees. Hence this recognitions is difficult to be achieved.

9. Altruistic Service than pursuit of material gain

There is a violation of this value and since there is no licensing, it does not affect the professional status of an HRD person.

The above discussion summarizes the following aspects in favor of recognizing HRD as a profession. They are:

- It has a body of knowledge which is highly contextual and more appropriate to today's society.
- It has professional bodies which needs to set and maintain standards, promote entry into the profession and establish and maintain professional standards.
- Has educational programs, though they need to be standardized.
- Has well defined roles and competencies.

In spite of a lot of developments in HRD, it is seen that

- The body of knowledge and the books do not outline the HRD applications in different contexts but restrict to the corporate sector, and hence serves only a small part of the population.
- There is no code of conduct, ethics and values for the profession.

- Professional bodies have shed away from formulating norms, values, certification requirements.
- There is no licensing mechanism.

We all know that professions like medicine and law have taken more than two centuries for acquiring the status of a profession after going through may stages of development. After judging against the criteria for a profession, it is seen that HRD in India, unlike the West has not been professionalized as it ought to be. HRD is an emerging field and would in future develop into a full fledged profession.

PROBLEMS AND ISSUES IN HRD

There are many problems faced by organizations with respect to HRD practices. These problems can be categorized into organizational and general problems.

Organizational Problems:

1. The top management of the organization often presume that by sending the managers to HRD programmes will automatically improve their performance, which is not a fact.
2. The managers do not show interest in developing the human resources. They argue that developing the human resources is the duty of the HRD department, which is a hindrance in the process of HRD.
3. There is a lack of genuine support to HRD programmes as they involve heavy expenditure
4. Most of the HRD department personnel do not have adequate training in HRD practices and process. This affects the HRD programmes.

General Problems

1. The HRD programmes fail due to poverty, social injustice, low quality education and illiteracy. The expected and required talents cannot be expected when employees are not financially well
2. The differences in religious faith among the people is also an hurdle for HRD. Many religious conflicts hinder development of HR.

3. Political interventions influences the moral behavior and development of right attitude and skills of HR in India.
4. The high population growth adversely affects the qualitative and quantitative dimensions of HRD programmes. High dependent population and unemployment add up the problems of HRD. This results in low per capita income, low savings and low investments. This downward shift in human resource status like health, education becomes inevitable.
5. The widening gap between the haves and the have nots is a hurdle in HRD. As Nehru said, "you cannot teach philosophy to a hungry person".
6. The strong faith in traditional methods which are linked with their religious philosophies generates a strong resistance to change and impairs the HRD process.

These problems could be overcome if the to management develops positive strategies.

The major issues and challenges facing the HRD today are:

Today Globalization is the greatest issue in HRD. The Indian economy has become an integral part of the global economy. Globalization means facing the competition and producing products and offering services of world standard quality. Total Quality Management, latest technology, sophisticated equipments, most up-to-date know-how, high skill, cost consciousness, production with less cost and customer's satisfaction have become the hallmarks for organizations to compete with others. In such a competitive environment, with the liberalization and globalization process of the economy, the organization will have to initiate radical changes within the organization to enable it to compete effectively. The HRD should act as catalyst to the changes required. HRD should ensure that every employee knows that they matter as an individual and a human being while the employer will have the confidence that the workforce will perform to the levels needed and beyond for success in today's competitive world. Hence HRD should handle human resource through training, education, job rotation, and reassignment. There is a need that a healthy climate, characterized by the values of openness, enthusiasm, mutuality, trust and collaboration be created for developing human resources.

The rapid changes in technology; and the emergence of more sophisticated and demanding consumers have brought about a proliferation of new and improved products. It has changed the customer perception. The use of information technologies has affected the organizational structure.

The greatest issue and challenge in organizations today is speed. The very survival of organizations become challenged, by the introduction of a new technology or a new computer. HR should voluntarily reassess its infrastructure and eliminate unnecessary rules and systems so that it can emphasize the need for individual judgment and accountability by administrators. This reassessment can be a powerful catalyst toward enabling organizational speed, creating change, and encouraging risk-taking.

Many HR functions and personnel are showing signs of insecurity, lack of identity and justification within their organization. HR personnel play a supporting role to the main objective of the organization, and therefore need to deliver something that contributes to the overall value. The reduced revenue is posing a great challenge to the current existence to the organizations. This has lead to cutbacks in terms of budgets, resources, equipment or layouts.

HR personnel should seek ways and means to measure its effectiveness and demonstrate its contribution to organizational profitability.

HR practitioners are presently under increasing pressures to rationalize operations resulting in reduction in workforce, and in restructuring of the organization and reduce dependence on specialists. The Department is often accused of being bureaucratic and reactive, but not responsive and objective oriented. They are also portrayed as slow and cumbersome even if they are not so in reality. They have to champion the existing innovative people initiatives.

Today's organizations, whether private or public sector, need to be flexible and competitive. Hence the traditional hierarchical structures are to be replaced by teams to meet the requirements of the organizations and achieve its objectives. When organizations are undergoing this change, the HRD not only needs to take part in the change, but also should play a key role in the process.

HRD needs to help in creating a powerful change by providing opportunities for the organization to identify its weakness, and facilitate organizational efforts to improve.

The principal issue for HRD in future is managing of education and skills training which has to be designed and delivered by subject matter experts or other managers but not by HR professionals alone. Majority of the organizations face the scarcity of principled leadership. Such leadership need to exist at all levels in an organization, and not just at top levels.

In future, the principal issue of HRD will be to focus on how its function can transform its outlook form a traditional to a modern one: from being functionally oriented, internally focused, reactive, activity driven, centralized, and control-oriented to being organization business oriented, customer focused, proactive, effectiveness drive, decentralized and empowerment oriented.

According to Dave Ulrich, HR will have to play four roles

First, strategic partner role-tuning strategy into results by building organizations that create value;

Second, a change agent role-making change happen and, in particular, help it happen fast;

The third, an employee champion role-managing the talent or the intellectual capital within an organization; and

The fourth, an administrative role-trying to get things happen better, faster and cheaper.

Organizations must focus on target groups and meet customer requirements. HR should eliminate policies and practices which prevent an external focus on the customer. HR should focus on the primacy of customer in every aspect of management practice by including customer orientation and customer service in performance reviews, promotion criteria and incentive compensation plans.

To overcome these challenges and the major issues today, the HRD must :

- eliminate HR systems and policies which inhibit speed in organizations.
- Focus on organization, rather than the job
- Support group performance rather than individual performance
- Be egalitarian and not hierarchical
- Change and not be stable
- Participate rather than command and control
- Develop principled leaders at all levels of the organization.
- Eliminate the HR's role in conducting training and education, by giving that role to subject experts and managers.
- Eliminate non-value added HR activities and outsource those HR activities which are not core competencies of the enterprise
- Increase the organization's ability to learn and collaborate, and to manage diversity, complexity, and ambiguity.

The HRD is under continuous challenge to its existence and needs to change to meet the new organizational needs.

The major issue before HRD is to find out the various factors which affect HRN at both national and regional levels so that appropriate human resource practices and policies can be formulated and successfully implemented.

The philosophy that human resource professionals should follow is : if you want to succeed you should strike out to new paths rather than travel the worn out paths of accepted success (John Rockfeller).

HRD EVALUATION

Periodic evaluation of how the HRD systems are working, whether the most appropriate practices are being used, can go a long way in resetting HRD and in realigning HRD to the organization's needs. There is need to evaluate and align or realign HRD continuously for organizational effectiveness. Without such periodic evaluation and realignment the HR function looses its credibility and place in the organization. This evaluation should be with respect to systems requirements, examining the competencies of HR people and the appropriateness of HR structures. It should also examine the quality of culture, working styles and behaviors created by HR practices. In short HRD should be evaluated in terms of its strategy, systems, structure and competencies, styles and culture it has developed in its employees.

There are various approaches for HRD evaluation. One such approach is the Integrative Framework.

The Integrative Framework: The Integrative Framework has been proposed by Yeung and Berman (1997). This framework identifies three paths through which HR practices can contribute to performance.

1. by building organizational capabilities
2. by improving employee satisfaction
3. by shaping customer and shareholder satisfaction.

This forms the first linkage chain. The second linkage chain which consists of organizational capabilities contributes to shareholder satisfaction. By evaluating these three paths and the organizational competencies the HRD can be evaluated.

Another approach can be through developing a HRD Score Card. The Score Card may be a 5 point or a 7 point rating scale where different aspects of HRD are rated. The different aspects of HRD that are to be rated include:

- HRD mechanisms or systems maturity
- Competencies of HRD staff
- Degree of HRD culture and HR competencies
- Alignment of HRD systems, competencies and culture with organizational goals.

HRD effectiveness depends on the above mentioned four indices. These four indices could be rated on either a 5 point or a 7 point scale. HRD audit can help in arriving at a HRD Score Card. HRD alignment or realignment can be possible through the information provided by HRD audit and HRD Score Card thus helping in building competitive people and processes.

HRD Evaluation

HRD Evaluation refers to an examination and evaluation of policies, procedures, and practices to determine the effectiveness of HRD. Before looking into HRD evaluation, let us try to understand the terms effectiveness and evaluation.

Effectiveness

- The degree to which HRD achieves its intended purpose
- Measures are relative to some starting point
- Measures how well the desired goal is achieved

Evaluation

Definition of HRD Evaluation

"The systematic collection of descriptive and judgmental information necessary to make effective HRD decisions related to the selection, adoption, value, and modification of various HRD activities."

The Evaluation needs to be undertaken as a proactive, creative, exercise with open participation by members of the function plus a representative sample of Personnel's internal clients. HRD evaluation is an essential step towards improving departmental credibility and overall quality goals.

The HRD evaluation is based on the premise that HR processes are dynamic and must continually be redirected and revitalized to remain responsive to the ever changing needs. It helps in providing insights into possible causes for current and future problems. HRD evaluation is also a systematic formal process, which is designed to examine the strategies, policies, procedures, documentation, structure, systems and practices.

The evaluation also reviews how well HR personnel comply with HR policies and procedures. The evaluation can improve HR department's image and contribution. The evaluation should cover three areas:

- Identifying current procedure and practice
- Analyzing cost and effectiveness of time and resource allocation
- Reviewing client's satisfaction and expectation.

It will help in highlighting the strength's and weaknesses and thus will identify areas for improvement.

HR practice and procedures are examined under the following broad categories of activities:

- Human resource strategy and planning
- Recruitment and selection
- Personnel records
- Salaries and remuneration
- Performance appraisal and review
- Training and development
- Policy and absenteeism
- Employee relations

Evaluation Needs

- Descriptive and judgmental information needed
- Objective and subjective data
- Information gathered according to a plan and in a desired format
- Gathered to provide decision making information

Purposes of Evaluation

- Determine whether the HRD is meeting the intended objectives
- Identify strengths and weaknesses
- Determine cost-benefit ratio
- Identify who benefited most or least
- Determine future participants
- Provide information for improving HRD programs
- Reinforce major points to be made
- Gather marketing information
- Determine if training program is appropriate
- Establish management database

Evaluation Bottom Line

- Is HRD a revenue contributor or a revenue user?
- Is HRD credible to line and upper-level managers?
- Are benefits of HRD readily evident to all?

Why HRD Evaluations are Rare

- Reluctance to having HRD programs evaluated
- Evaluation needs expertise and resources

Factors other than HRD cause performance improvements – e.g.,

- Economy
- Equipment
- Policies, etc.

Need for HRD Evaluation

- Shows the value of HRD
- Provides metrics for HRD efficiency
- Demonstrates value-added approach for HRD
- Demonstrates accountability for HRD activities
- Everyone else has it... why not HRD?

Evolution of Evaluation Efforts

1. *Anecdotal* approach – talk to other users
2. *Try before buy* – borrow and use samples
3. *Analytical* approach – match research data to training needs
4. *Holistic* approach – look at overall HRD process, as well as individual training

For evaluation of HRD, firstly the existing data has to be collected, such as, hiring statistics, compensation practice, exist interview, summaries, employee complaints, human resource budget and expenditures. Secondly, interviews have to be conducted to collect input from the internal customer on their human resources needs and how those needs are being met. It has to begin with top management and then percolate down.

Data Collection for HRD Evaluation Possible methods:

Interviews

Advantages

- Flexible
- Opportunity for clarification
- Depth possible
- Personal contact

Limitations

- High reactive effects
- High cost
- Face-to-face threat potential
- Labor intensive
- Trained observers needed

Questionnaires

Advantages

- Low cost to administer
- Honesty increased
- Anonymity possible
- Respondent sets the pace
- Variety of options

Limitations

- Possible inaccurate data
- Response conditions not controlled
- Respondents set varying paces
- Uncontrolled return rate

Direct observation

Advantages

- Non-threatening
- Excellent way to measure behavior change

Limitations

- Possibly disruptive
- Reactive effects are possible
- May be unreliable
- Need trained observers

Written tests

Advantages

- Low purchase cost
- Readily scored
- Quickly processed
- Easily administered
- Wide sampling possible

Limitations

- May be threatening
- Possibly no relation to job performance
- Measures only cognitive learning
- Relies on norms
- Concern for racial/ ethnic bias

Simulation/Performance tests

Advantages

- Reliable
- Objective
- Close relation to job performance
- Includes cognitive, psychomotor and affective domains

Limitations

- Time consuming
- Simulations often difficult to create
- High costs to development and use

Archival performance information

Advantages

- Reliable

- Objective
- Job-based
- Easy to review
- Minimal reactive effects

Limitations

- Criteria for keeping/ discarding records
- Information system discrepancies
- Indirect
- Not always usable
- Records prepared for other purposes

Choosing Data Collection Methods

- Reliability
    - Consistency of results, and freedom from collection method bias and error
- Validity
    - Does the device measure what we want to measure?
- Practicality
    - Does it make sense in terms of the resources used to get the data?

Type of Data Used/Needed

- Individual performance
- System wide performance
- Economic

Individual Performance Data

- Individual knowledge
- Individual behaviors

Examples:

- Test scores
- Performance quantity, quality, and timeliness
- Attendance records
- Attitudes

System wide Performance Data

- Productivity
- Scrap/rework rates
- Customer satisfaction levels
- On-time performance levels
- Quality rates and improvement rates

Economic Data

- Profits
- Product liability claims
- Avoidance of penalties
- Market share
- Competitive position
- Return on investment (ROI)
- Financial utility calculations

Ways to Improve HRD Assessment

- Walk the walk, talk the talk: MONEY
- Involve HRD in strategic planning
- Involve management in HRD planning and estimation efforts
- Gain mutual ownership
    - Use credible and conservative estimates
    - Share credit for successes and blame for failures

HRD Evaluation Steps

1. Analyze needs.
2. Determine explicit evaluation strategy.
3. Insist on specific and measurable training objectives.
4. Obtain participant reactions.
5. Develop criterion measures/instruments to measure results.
6. Plan and execute evaluation strategy.

The primary purpose of HRD evaluation is to know how the various units are functioning and how they have been able to meet the policies and guidelines which are agreed upon; and to assist the rest of the organization by identifying the gap between objectives and results, for the end-product of an evaluation should be to formulate plans for corrections or adjustments.

The main benefits of HRD evaluation are :

1. it identifies the contribution of personnel to the organization
2. it improves the professional image of HRD
3. it encourages greater responsibility of professionalism among members of HRD
4. it promotes uniformity of personnel policies and practices
5. it helps to locate key personnel problem areas
6. it ensures timely compliance of statutory requirements
7. it helps to reduce personnel costs by proper utilization of human resources
8. it brings about desirable changes in the functioning of HRD.

The specific evaluation questions that could be raised in assessing the benefits and services accruing from HRD are:

- Is the manpower planning in consonance with the overall plan of the organization?
- Is the recruitment and selection process effective in tracing the individual knowledge, skills and aptitude at the initial stage?
- How effective is the orientation programme in inducting the new employees to company policies, procedures and goals?
- Whether the performance appraisal system is effective in identifying the strengths and weaknesses of their employees and their development needs?
- How effective are the training, development, and career planning activities in preparing people for selection and placement into the present and future positions in the organization?
- How are the training needs identified, knowledge and skill imparted and benefits evaluated?
- How effective are the reward systems - both financial and non-financial - in motivating individual employees?
- What is the role of participative mechanism in developing the organization and its human resource?

- What is the state of prevailing organizational climate and employee morale in the organization?

Conducting an HRD evaluation is the first and crucial step in improving the service of HRD. It collects facts and evidence of what is actually done and what needs to be done. The evaluation also helps HRD to clarify its role and sets out the priorities for action. The department can assess which actions will lead to most benefits in terms of improved value to the organization. It gives feedback about the HR function to managers and HR specialists. In short, HRD evaluation is quality control check on HR activities. It reminds HR personnel of the departments contribution and creates a more professional image of the department among the personnel and HR specialists. It also helps to clarify the department's role and leads to greater uniformity. An effective HRD meets both company objectives and employee needs.

SUMMARY

Concerns about professionalism and professionalization of HRD have been in existence since the last decade. The issue of professionalizing HRD was taken up by the National HRD Network in their symposium in 1990. Based on the core criteria of a profession, HRD can be identified as a profession today. We all know that professions like medicine and law have taken more than two centuries for acquiring the status of a profession after going through may stages of development. After judging against the criteria for a profession, it is seen that HRD in India, unlike the West has not been professionalized as it ought to be. HRD is an emerging field and would in future develop into a full fledged profession.

Basically, the professionals in the Personnel department are considered "staff" rather than "line" personnel since they provide specialized advice to the production or operations mangers. Their function consists of advising, developing and administering policies and programmes affecting human resources. In addition to specific functions in the area of employment, safety and training, the personnel department is responsible for research and advice regarding personnel policies and procedures, facilitation of internal communication, administration of benefit schemes and community relations.

The role of Personnel management is to plan, develop, and administer policies and programmes designed to make expeditious use of an organization's resources.

There are many problems faced by organizations with respect to HRD practices. These problems can be categorized into organizational and general problems. Today Globalization, Total Quality Management, latest technology, sophisticated equipments, most up-to-date know-how, high skill, cost consciousness, production with less cost, customer's satisfaction, liberalization and globalization process of the economy, the rapid changes in technology, the emergence of more sophisticated and demanding consumers, speed, the reduced revenue is posing a great challenge to the current existence to the organizations.

Periodic evaluation of how the HRD systems are working, whether the most appropriate practices are being used, can go a long way in resetting HRD and in realigning HRD to the organization's needs. There is need to evaluate and align or realign HRD continuously for organizational effectiveness. Without such periodic evaluation and realignment the HR function looses its credibility and place in the organization. This evaluation should be with respect to systems requirements, examining the competencies of HR people and the appropriateness of HR structures. It should also examine the quality of culture, working styles and behaviors created by HR practices. In short HRD should be evaluated in terms of its strategy, systems, structure and competencies, styles and culture it has developed in its employees. There are various approaches for HRD evaluation. HRD evaluation is the systematic collection of descriptive and judgmental information necessary to make effective HRD decisions related to the selection, adoption, value, and modification of various HRD activities. HRD must justify itself repeatedly as a revenue enhancer.

UNIT 9

COUNSELLING IN HUMAN RESOURCE DEVELOPMENT

INTRODUCTION

Counselling

Counselling is called the crux, heart, essence, pivot or core of all the programmes. The proper functioning and growth of the body depends upon the proper functioning of the heart. Similarly, the success or failure of any programme is determined by the counselling service. One who performs the functions of guidance is called a counsellor. The word Counsellor is derived from the word 'Counsel' which means advice or help. A Counsellor is one who is "trained" to offer help to a person who face problems that they can not solve for themselves. The trust or confidence a Counsellor has toward a counselee is termed Rapport.

Process of Counselling in HRD

The counselling process has three phases:

- Rapport building
- Exploration
- Action Planning

Rapport Building: in this phase, a good counselor attempts to establish a climate of acceptance, warmth, support, openness and mutuality. This phase involves generating confidence in the employee to open up and frankly share his perceptions, problems, concerns, feelings etc. the subordinate must be made to feel that he is wanted and that his superior is genuinely interested in his development

Exploration: after establishing a climate of openness and trust and listening to the employee, the superior should attempt to help the employee understand and appreciate his strengths and weaknesses. He should also understand his own situation, problems and needs. Counseling skill lies in making the employee to discover these on his own so that he is motivated to take remedial measures enthusiastically.

This can be achieved through asking questions which help the employee focus on his problem. For example: if an employee is facing problems with adjusting to his colleagues, the superior may ask questions to help the employee understand what is causing adjustment problems to him. Problem identification is a critical step in planning for improvement. Diagnosis of the problem should follow exploration. Here the efforts should generate several alternative causes of a problem. Open ended questions may help the employee to make a correct diagnosis of the problem. Questions like, " At what instances do you think you did not have any adjustment problems with your colleagues".

Action Planning: Counseling interviews should end with specific plans of action for the development of the employee. The main contribution of the superior in this phase is helping the employee think of alternative ways of dealing with a problem. For example he can ask, "what three things can you do in the next week to improve your adjustment with your colleagues?" After helping the employee brainstorm, the superior may also add some more alternatives to the solutions already generated. However, the primary responsibility of generating the solutions must be with the employee himself. After alternative solutions to the performance problem have been identified, the superior should help the employee to assess the advantages and disadvantages of each. Finally the superior may render some assistance in helping the employee implement the agreed upon action plan.

Questions play an important role in performance counseling. They can help ingathering more information, stimulating thinking and directing the employee towards solutions to problems. However, if questions are not asked in a proper manner they may even hinder communication. Hence the framing of the questions, the tone in which it is delivered, and the situation in which it is delivered play a vital role. Critical, testing and leading questions hinder communication

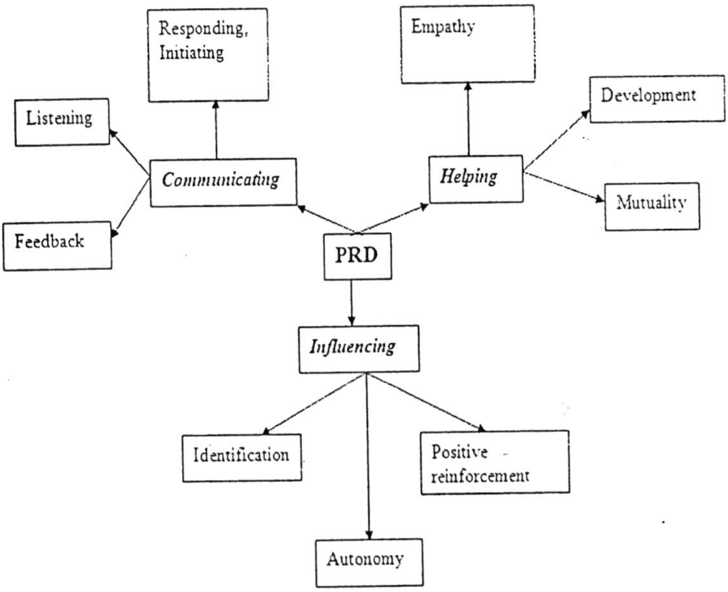

Fig 9.1: The Process of PRD Empathy

whereas open empathetic questions facilitate communication. Paraphrasing questions enable the superior to verify that he has correctly heard and understood the subordinate. The process of Performance counseling or performance review discussion is as depicted in the Fig. 9.1.

Listening is the first effective step in communication. It involves paying attention to the various messages being sent by the other person. Responding to questions and feelings are also an important part of communication. Feedback is an important part of PRD.

It is extremely important that feedback is communicated in a manner that produces a constructive response in the subordinate. Most of the superiors find it extremely embarrassing to provide negative feedback. Feedback is effective if the person who is providing feedback makes sure that it is

- descriptive and non-evaluative.
- focused on the behavior of the person and not on the person himself. It should be clear to the employee that what is being

rejected or criticized is some specific behavior of his. The intent is not condemning the employee as an individual. This can be achieved by being fairly specific in pointing out to the employee the behavior patterns that need corrective action.

- data-based and not impressionistic. When conveying feedback, it is desirable to show some examples of actual events.
- suggestive not prescriptive so that the subordinate is kept in a receptive frame of mind.
- timely.
- continuous. It should be a regular practice so that the subordinate develops an ability to accept and act upon feedback
- checked and verified since it ensures that the subordinate has not interpreted the feedback he has received form his superior
- reinforcing positive behavior. The superior should acknowledge any improvement he perceives in the subordinate's behavior so that old patterns are replaced and reinforced by new ones.
- need based and solicited.
- intended to help.
- focused on modifiable behavior.
- satisfies the needs of both the superior and the subordinate.

Performance counseling is an effective mechanism for individual and organizational development, and learning and its effectiveness in that regard will depend on factors like designed questions, preparedness of rater and rater, and the organization.

JOB ENRICHMENT

You know that retaining experienced employees is a key factor in an organization's success. Organizations cannot afford to lose these people to competition from other organizations. If the root causes of the scenarios are truly related to boredom and lack of preparation for advancement, job enrichment could be an excellent non-training intervention. One technique to retain experienced employees and to motivate them in the present job is Job enrichment.

Job enrichment is an attempt to *motivate* employees by giving them the opportunity to use the range of their abilities. It is an idea that was developed by the American *psychologist Frederick Herzberg* in the 1950s.

Job Enrichment is the addition to a job of tasks that increase the amount of employee control or responsibility. It is a vertical expansion of the job as opposed to the horizontal expansion of a job, which is called job enlargement. Job enrichment is used to make work more challenging and rewarding for employees to make it easier to keep them.

It can be contrasted to *job enlargement* which simply increases the number of tasks without changing the challenge. As such job enrichment has been described as 'vertical loading' of a job, while job enlargement is 'horizontal loading'. An enriched job should ideally contain:

- A range of tasks and challenges of varying difficulties
- A complete unit of work - a meaningful task
- Feedback, encouragement and communication

Job enrichment is a type of job redesign intended to reverse the effects of tasks that are repetitive requiring little autonomy. Some of these effects are boredom, lack of flexibility, and employee dissatisfaction (Leach & Wall, 2004). The underlying principle is to expand the scope of the job with a greater variety of tasks, vertical in nature, that require self-sufficiency. Since the goal is to give the individual exposure to tasks normally reserved for differently focused or higher positions, merely adding more of the same responsibilities related to an employee's current position is not considered job enrichment.

Job enrichment is a way to motivate employees by giving them increased responsibility and variety in their jobs. Many employers traditionally believed that money was the only true motivating factor for employees and that if you wanted to get more work out of employees, offering them more money was the only way to do it. While that may be true for a small group of people, the majority of workers today like to work and to be appreciated for the work they do. Job enrichment—allowing the employees to have more control in planning their work and deciding how the work should be accomplished—is one way to tap into the natural desire most employees have to do a good job, to be appreciated for their contributions to the company, and to feel more a part of the company team.

Job enrichment has its roots in Frederick Herzberg's *two-factor theory*, according to which two separate dimensions contribute to an employee's behavior at work. The first dimension, known as hygiene factors, involves the presence or absence of job dissatisfacters, such as wages, working environment, rules and regulations, and supervisors. When these factors are poor, work is dissatisfying and employees are not motivated. However, having positive hygiene factors does not cause employees to be motivated; it simply keeps them from being dissatisfied. The second dimension of Herzberg's theory refers to motivators, which are factors that satisfy higher-level needs such as recognition for doing a good job, achievement, and the opportunity for growth and responsibility. These motivators are what actually increase job satisfaction and performance. Job enrichment becomes an important strategy at this point because enriching employees' jobs can help meet some of their motivational needs. There are basically five areas that are believed to affect an individual employee's motivation and job performance: skill variety, task identity, task significance, autonomy, and feedback. Job enrichment seeks to find positive ways to address each of these areas and therefore improve employee motivation and personal satisfaction.

Skill variety involves the number of different types of skills that are used to do a job. This area is important because using only one skill to do the same task repeatedly can be quite boring, typically causing the employee's productivity to decrease after a period of time. However, using a variety of skills in a job will tend to keep the employee more interested in the job and more motivated.

One way businesses are focusing on this area is through *job rotation*, that is, moving employees from job to job within the company, thereby allowing employees a variety of tasks in their work and helping prevent boredom. While this process can be costly to the company because employees must be trained in several different areas, the cost tends to be balanced by the increase in morale and productivity. Job rotation also gives each employee the opportunity to see how the different jobs of a company fit together and gives the company more flexibility in covering tasks when workers are absent. However, while job rotation is a good way to enrich employees' jobs, it can also hinder performance: Having to know several different jobs in order to rotate, can prevent employees from becoming proficient at any of the jobs. Therefore, the advantages and disadvantages of job rotation as an enrichment strategy have to be carefully weighed.

Task identity is a matter of realizing a visible outcome from performing a task. Being able to see the end result of the work they do is an important motivator for employees. One way to make task identity clearer is through *job enlargement*, which means adding more tasks and responsibilities to an existing job. For example, instead of building just one component part of a humidifier, a team of employees builds the entire product from start to finish. When using job enlargement as an enrichment strategy, it is important that enlarging the job gives the employee more responsibility and more variety, not just more work.

Task significance involves how important the task is to others in the company, which is important in showing employees how the work they do fits in with that done in the rest of the organization. If employees can see how their work affects others, it will be a motivator to do the best job they can.

Many companies take new employees on a tour of the company and provide training sessions on how each part of the company works together with the other parts. In order to accept and handle responsibility, it is important that employees know how the various areas of the company work together; without this knowledge, it is very difficult for them to handle decision-making responsibilities. Putting employees from different areas of the company into planning teams can also help them see the significance of the tasks they perform.

Autonomy involves the degree of freedom, independence, and decision-making ability the employee has in completing assigned tasks. Most people like to be given responsibility; it demonstrates trust and helps motivate employees to live up to that trust. Responsibility can also help speed up work processes by enabling the employee to make decisions without having to wait for management approval. Autonomy is a very important part of job enrichment because it gives the employee power and a feeling of importance.

A type of job enrichment that restructures work to best match the employee to the job is *job redesign*. Job redesign can focus on combining existing jobs, forming work groups, and/or allowing closer contact between employees and individual suppliers or customers. The idea behind job redesign is to match employees with a job they like and are best qualified to perform. Self-managed teams are a type of job design whereby employees are grouped into teams and given certain guidelines to follow as well as goals to accomplish—and then left alone to accomplish those goals. Self-managed teams demonstrate the company's faith in the employees and give employees a feeling of power and pride in the work they accomplish.

Feedback describes how much and what type of information about job performance is received by the employee. It is one of the most important areas for motivation. Without feedback, employees have no way of knowing whether they are doing things correctly or incorrectly. Positive feedback helps to motivate employees by recognizing the efforts they have put into their work. While monetary rewards for doing a good job can be a strong incentive, sometimes saying "you did a really good job on that project" can mean just as much. Corrective feedback is also important because it lets employees know what areas need improvement.

Job enrichment, as a managerial activity includes ***a three steps technique***:

1. Turn employees' effort into performance:

- Ensuring that objectives are well-defined and understood by everyone. The overall corporate *mission statement* should be communicated to all. Individual's goals should also be clear. Each employee should know exactly how he/she fits into the overall process and be aware of how important their contributions are to the organization and its customers.

- Providing adequate resources for each employee to perform well. This includes support functions like information technology, communication technology, and personnel training and development.
- Creating a supportive corporate culture. This includes peer support networks, supportive management, and removing elements that foster mistrust and politicking.
- Free flow of information. Eliminate secrecy.
- Provide enough freedom to facilitate job excellence. Encourage and reward employee initiative. Flextime or compressed hours could be offered.
- Provide adequate recognition, appreciation, and other motivators.
- Provide skill improvement opportunities. This could include paid education at universities or on the job training.
- Provide job variety. This can be done by job sharing or job rotation programmes.
- It may be necessary to re-engineer the job process. This could involve redesigning the physical facility, redesign processes, change technologies, simplification of procedures, elimination of repetitiveness, redesigning authority structures.

2. Link employees performance directly to reward:

- Clear definition of the reward is a must
- Explanation of the link between performance and reward is important
- Make sure the employee gets the right reward if performs well
- If reward is not given, explanation is needed

3. Make sure the employee wants the reward. How to find out?

- Ask them
- Use surveys(checklist, listing, questions)

The work done by Frederick Herzberg in the 1950's and 60's, was further refined in 1975 by Hackman and Oldham using what they called the Job Characteristics Model. This model assumes that if five core job characteristics are present, three psychological states critical to motivation are produced, resulting in positive outcomes (Kotila, 2001). Fig. 9.2 illustrates this model.

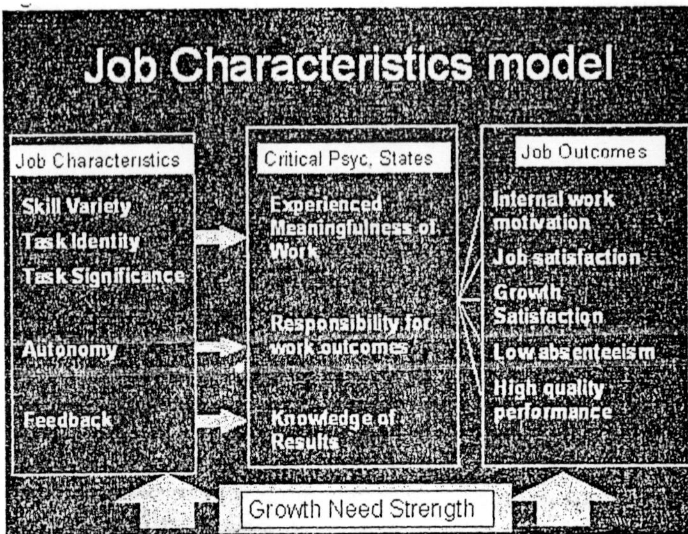

Note. From Drez, J. (1999). *Chapter seven motivation through needs, job design, and satisfaction, slide 20.* Retrieved February 14, 2004, from http://www.siu.edu/departments/cola/psych/psyc323/chat07/index.htm.

Fig. 9.2

Job enrichment can only be truly successful if planning includes support for all phases of the initiative. Ohio State University Extension began a job enrichment program in 1992 and surveyed the participants five years later. The results, broken down into 3 sub-buckets of data beyond the main grouping of advantages/disadvantages, indicate the

Figure 2: Ohio State University Extension Job Enrichment Survey Results

ADVANTAGES	Renewal:	reduction in boredom, making new contacts, thinking about new career options, change in viewpoint.
	Exploration:	trying new skills, developing new relationships, testing management & administrative skills.
	Specialization:	re-education, in-depth exploration, using special skills, meeting a need that was under-served.
DISADVANTAGES	Balance:	time allocation, tough decisions about work load, taking time away from regular assignments, balancing work load.
	Clarity:	lack of information needed to be successful, lack of clear plans and goals, guidance in using time.
	Orientation:	lack of structured introduction to special assignment, not being taught new responsibilities, difficulty in learning new networks, lack of instruction, sink or swim approach.

Note. The data represented are from "Job Enrichment in Extension," by Louis S. Fourman and Jo Jones, 1997, *Journal of Extension, 35*, Retrieved February 14, 2004, from http://www.joe.org/joe/1997october/iw1.html

University had not fully considered the planning and administrative aspects of the program (Fourman and Jones, 1997). While the benefits are seemingly obvious, programs fail not because of a lack of benefits, but rather due to implementation problems. These problems can include a perception of too great a cost, lack of long-term commitment of resources, and potential job classification changes (Cunningham and Eberle, 1990).

In order for a job enrichment program to produce positive results, worker needs and organizational needs must be analyzed and acted upon. According to Cunningham and Eberle (1990), before an enrichment program is begun, the following questions should be asked:

1. Do employees need jobs that involve responsibility, variety, feedback, challenge, accountability, significance, and opportunities to learn?
2. What techniques can be implemented without changing the job classification plan?
3. What techniques would require changes in the job classification plan?

There are many different types of job-enrichment activities and programs that companies can implement to encourage worker participation and enhance motivation. The team atmosphere is one way to enrich jobs. Grouping employees into teams and allowing the team the freedom to plan, make decisions, and accomplish their goals gives employees a feeling of importance and responsibility. It can also help employees come up with creative ideas on ways to improve work activities by giving them the opportunity to work closely with others. Asking for and encouraging employees to give input on company strategies and plans is another way to enrich jobs. Often times employees have the best input because they are the ones actually performing the activity on a daily basis. Holding company award ceremonies can also help to enrich jobs and motivate employees by recognizing individual employees for their contributions to the company.

The purpose of job enrichment is to improve the quality of an employee's job and therefore motivate the employee to accomplish more. However, in order for job enrichment to work, the employee has to desire and accept new ways of accomplishing tasks. Some employees lack the skills and knowledge required to perform enriched jobs, while others are quite happy doing routine jobs because they feel the current work situation is relatively stress-free. It is likely that these types of employees would not like job-enrichment activities and would not accept the new way of doing things. Therefore, asking for employee input and keeping communication lines open is essential to the success of job-enrichment programs.

QUALITY OF WORKING LIFE

Quality of life and Quality of work are closely interrelated. Fig. 9.3 depicts this relationship.

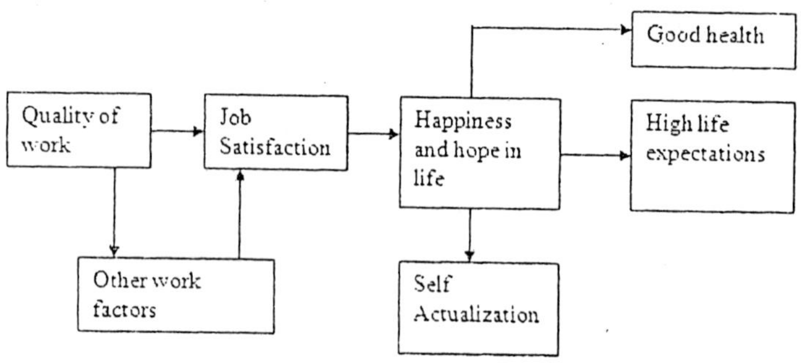

Fig: 9.3 : Relationship of Quality of life and Quality of work

Quality of Working Life is a term that had been used to describe the broader *job*-related experience an individual has.

Quality of Working Life refers to the *"degree to which work provides an opportunity for an individual to satisfy a wide variety of personal needs from the need to survive with some security to the need to interact with others, to have a sense of personal usefulness, to be recognized for achievement, and to have an opportunity to improve one's skills and knowledge".*

A large chunk of most peoples' lives will be spent at work. Most people recognise the importance of sleeping well, and actively try to enjoy the leisure time that they can snatch. But all too often, people tend to see work as something they just have to put up with, or even something they don't even expect to enjoy.

Some of the factors used to measure quality of working life pick up on things that don't actually make people feel good, but which seem to make people feel bad about work if those things are absent. For example, noise – if the place where someone works is too noisy, they might get frequent headaches, or find they can not concentrate, and so feel dissatisfied. But when it is quiet enough they don't feel pleased or happy - they just don't feel bad. This can apply to a range of factors that affect someone's working conditions.

Other things seem to be more likely to make people feel good about work and themselves once the basics are OK at work. Challenging work (not too little, not too much) can make them feel good. Similarly, opportunities for career progression and using their abilities can contribute to someone's quality of working life.

While there has, for many years, been much research into job satisfaction, more recently, an interest has arisen into the broader concepts of stress and subjective well-being, the precise nature of the relationship between these concepts has still been little explored. Stress at work is often considered in isolation, wherein it is assessed on the basis that attention to an individual's stress management skills or the sources of stress will prove to provide a good enough basis for effective intervention. Alternatively, job satisfaction may be assessed, so that action can be taken which will enhance an individual's performance. Somewhere in all this, there is often an awareness of the greater context, whereupon the home-work context is considered, for example, and other factors, such as an individual's personal characteristics, and the broader economic or cultural climate, might be seen as relevant. In this context, subjective well-being is seen as drawing upon both work and non-work aspects of life.

However, more complex models of an individuals experience in the workplace often appear to be set aside in an endeavour to simplify the process of trying to measuring "stress" or some similarly apparently discrete entity. It may be, however, that the consideration of the bigger, more complex picture is essential, if targeted, effective action is to be taken to address quality of working life or any of it's sub-components in such a way as to produce real benefits, be they for the individual or the organisation.

Quality of working life has been differentiated from the broader concept of Quality of Life. To some degree, this may be overly simplistic, as Elizur and Shye (1990) concluded that quality of work performance is affected by Quality of Life as well as Quality of working life. This consideration of Quality of working Life as the greater context for various factors in the workplace, such as job satisfaction and stress, may offer opportunity for more cost-effective interventions in the workplace.

Various authors and researchers have proposed ***models of Quality of working life*** which include a wide range of factors. Selected models are given below:

Hackman and Oldham (1976) drew attention to what they described as psychological growth needs as relevant to the consideration of Quality of working life. Several such needs were identified; Skill variety, Task Identity, Task significance, Autonomy and Feedback. They suggested that such needs have to be addressed if employees are to experience high quality of working life.

In contrast to such theory based models, Taylor (1979) more pragmatically identified the essential components of Quality of working life as; basic extrinsic job factors of wages, hours and working conditions, and the intrinsic job notions of the nature of the work itself. He suggested that a number of other aspects could be added, including; individual power, employee participation in the management, fairness and equity, social support, use of one's present skills, self development, a meaningful future at work, social relevance of the work or product, effect on extra work activities. Taylor suggested that relevant Quality of working life concepts may vary according to organisation and employee group.

Warr and colleagues (1979), in an investigation of Quality of working life, considered a range of apparently relevant factors, including work involvement, intrinsic job motivation, higher order need strength, perceived intrinsic job characteristics, job satisfaction, life satisfaction, happiness, and self-rated anxiety. They discussed a range of correlations derived from their work, such as those between work involvement and job satisfaction, intrinsic job motivation and job satisfaction, and perceived intrinsic job characteristics and job satisfaction. In particular, Warr et al., found evidence for a moderate association between total job satisfaction and total life satisfaction and happiness, with a less strong, but significant association with self-rated anxiety.

Thus, while some authors have emphasised the workplace aspects in Quality of working life, others have identified the relevance of personality factors, psychological well being, and broader concepts of happiness and life satisfaction.

Factors affecting Quality of Working Life

Factors more obviously and directly affecting work have served as the main focus of attention, as researchers have tried to identify the important influences on Quality of working life in the workplace.

Mirvis and Lawler (1984) suggested that Quality of working life was associated with satisfaction with wages, hours and working conditions, describing the "basic elements of a good quality of work life" as; safe work environment, equitable wages, equal employment opportunities and opportunities for advancement.

Baba and Jamal (1991) listed what they described as typical indicators of quality of working life, including: job satisfaction, job involvement, work role ambiguity, work role conflict, work role overload, job stress, organisational commitment and turn-over intentions. Baba and Jamal also explored routinisation of job content, suggesting that this facet should be investigated as part of the concept of quality of working life.

Some have argued that quality of working life might vary between groups of workers. For example, Ellis and Pompli (2002) identified a number of factors contributing to job dissatisfaction and quality of working life in nurses, including: Poor working environments, Resident aggression, Workload, Unable to deliver quality of care preferred, Balance of work and family, Shiftwork, Lack of involvement in decision making, Professional isolation, Lack of recognition, Poor relationships with supervisor/peers, Role conflict, Lack of opportunity to learn new skills.

Sirgy et al. (2001) suggested that the key factors in quality of working life are: Need satisfaction based on job requirements, Need satisfaction based on Work environment, Need satisfaction based on Supervisory behaviour, Need satisfaction based on Ancillary programmes, Organizational commitment. They defined quality of working life as satisfaction of these key needs through resources, activities, and outcomes stemming from participation in the workplace. Maslow's needs were seen as relevant in underpinning this model, covering Health & safety, Economic and family, Social, Esteem, Actualisation, Knowledge and Aesthetics, although the relevance of non-work aspects is play down as attention is focussed on quality of work life rather than the broader concept of quality of life.

The attempts at defining quality of working life have included theoretical approaches, lists of identified factors, correlational analyses, with opinions varying as to whether such definitions and explanations can be both global, or need to be specific to each work setting.

Bearfield, (2003) used 16 questions to examine quality of working life, and distinguished between causes of dissatisfaction in professionals, intermediate clerical, sales and service workers, indicating that different concerns might have to be addressed for different groups.

The distinction made between job satisfaction and dissatisfaction in quality of working life reflects the influence of job satisfaction theories. Herzberg at al., (1959) used "Hygiene factors" and "Motivator factors" to distinguish between the separate causes of job satisfaction and job dissatisfaction. It has been suggested that Motivator factors are intrinsic to the job, that is; job content, the work itself, responsibility and advancement. The Hygiene factors or dissatisfaction-avoidance factors include aspects of the job environment such as interpersonal relationships, salary, working conditions and security. Of these latter, the most common cause of job dissatisfaction can be company policy and administration, whilst achievement can be the greatest source of extreme satisfaction.

An individual's experience of satisfaction or dissatisfaction can be substantially rooted in their perception, rather than simply reflecting their "real world". Further, an individual's perception can be affected by relative comparison – am I paid as much as that person - and comparisons of internalised ideals, aspirations, and expectations, for example, with the individual's current state (Lawler and Porter, 1966).

It has generally been agreed that Quality of Working Life is conceptually similar to well-being of employees but differs from job satisfaction which solely represents the workplace domain (Lawler, 1982).

Quality of Working Life is not a unitary concept, but has been seen as incorporating a hierarchy of perspectives that not only include work-based factors such as job satisfaction, satisfaction with pay and relationships with work colleagues, but also factors that broadly reflect life satisfaction and general feelings of well-being (Danna & Griffin, 1999). More recently, work-related stress and the relationship between work and non-work life domains (Loscocco & Roschelle, 1991) have also been identified as factors that should conceptually be included in Quality of Working Life.

Measurement of Quality of Working Life

There are few recognised measures of quality of working life, and of those that exist few have evidence of validity and reliability, that is, there is a very limited literature based on peer reviewed evaluations of available assessments. A recent statistical analysis of a new measure, the Work-Related Quality of Life scale (WRQoL), indicates that this assessment device should prove to be a useful instrument, although further evaluation would be useful. The WRQoL measure uses 6 core factors to explain most of the variation in an individuals quality of working life: Job and Career Satisfaction; Working Conditions; General Well-Being; Home-Work Interface; Stress at Work and Control at Work.

Regular assessment of Quality of Working Life can potentially provide organisations with important information about the welfare of their employees, such as job satisfaction, general well-being, work-related stress and the home-work interface.

Worrall and Cooper (2006) reported that a low level of well-being at work is estimated to cost about 5-10% of Gross National Product per annum, yet Quality of Working Life as a theoretical construct remains relatively unexplored and unexplained within the organisational psychology research literature.

The success of any organization is highly dependant on how it attracts, recruits, motivates, and retains its workforce. Today's organizations need to be more flexible so that they are equipped to develop their workforce and enjoy their commitment.

Therefore, organizations are required to adopt a strategy to improve the employees' 'quality of work life' (QWL) to satisfy both the organizational objectives and employee needs. Quality of work life practices in organizations have an impact on employee performance and the overall organizational performance.

HRD LINKAGES

1. Organizational Effectiveness Dimensions
2. HRD Outcomes Variables
3. HRD Process and HRD Climate Variables
4. HRD Mechanisms/Subsystems/Instruments

- Higher productivity
- Growth and diversification
- Cost reduction
- More profits
- Better image
- More competent people
- Better developed roles
- Higher work commitment and job involvement
- More problem solving
- Better utilization of human resources
- Higher job satisfaction and work motivation
- Better generation of internal resources
- Better organizational health

Figure 9.4 explains the linkages between HRD instruments, processes, outcomes and organizational effectiveness.

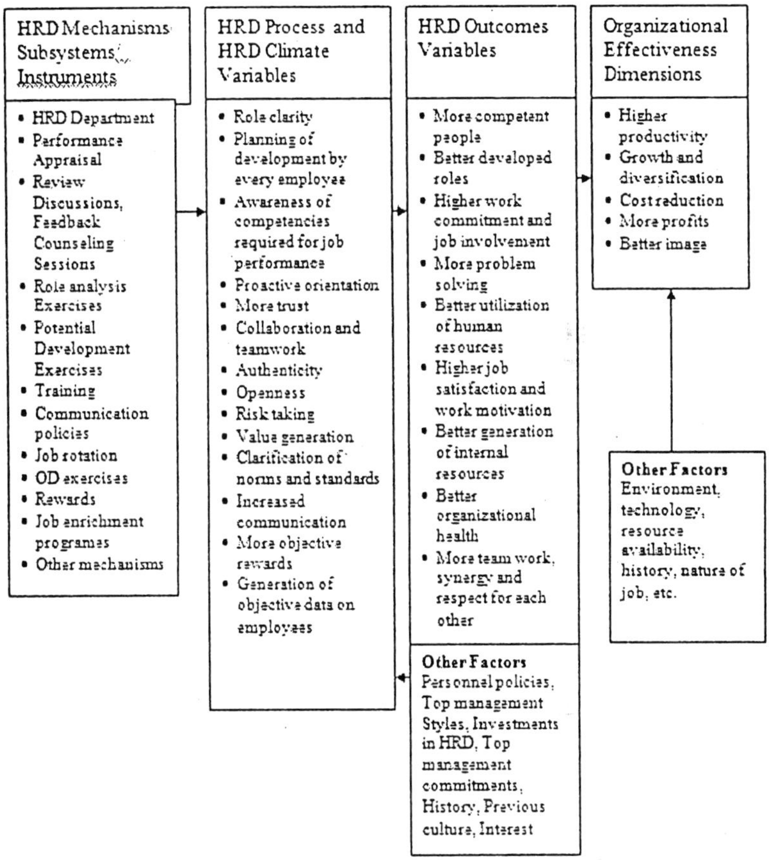

Fig. 9.4: Schematic representation of HRD Linkages

- More team work, synergy and respect for each other
- Role clarity
- Planning of development by every employee
- Awareness of competencies required for job performance
- Proactive orientation
- More trust
- Collaboration and teamwork
- Authenticity
- Openness

- Risk taking
- Value generation
- Clarification of norms and standards
- Increased communication
- More objective rewards
- Generation of objective data on employees
- HRD Department
- Performance Appraisal
- Review Discussions, Feedback Counseling Sessions
- Role analysis Exercises
- Potential Development Exercises
- Training
- Communication policies
- Job rotation
- OD exercises
- Rewards
- Job enrichment programmes
- Other mechanisms

Other Factors

- Environment, technology, resource availability, history, nature of job, etc.
- Personnel policies, Top management Styles, Investments in HRD, Top management commitments, History, Previous culture, Interest

The Fig. 9.4 depicts the linkages between HRD Instruments, Processes, Outcomes and Organizational effectiveness. *HRD instruments* are various tools of HRD that are used by organizations for building competence, commitment and culture. These tools include performance appraisal system, feedback and counseling, potential development exercises like training. These tools when used effectively will create a conducive HRD culture and HRD learning processes. The HRD process variables include role clarity, work planning, awareness of competencies, better communication and the practice of HRD values like openness, collaboration, trust, proaction authenticity, autonomy etc. These HRD culture and processes result in HRD outcomes like higher level of managerial, human relation and conceptual competencies, better utilization of human resources, higher work commitment work motivation, greater team work and synergy. These HRD outcomes greatly influence the effectiveness of working of the organization in terms of achievement of its goals, high productivity, cost reduction, better image and satisfied stake holders. This linkage between HRD variables will lead to good HRD practices that would help in building competencies and commitment of employees.

EDUCATION: THE DOMINANT HUMAN RESOURCE FACTOR

In the changing socio-economic and technological conditions, the human resource occupies a key position. Human resource refers to manpower resources. By human resources we mean total skill, knowledge, talents, creative ability and aptitudes of "People" in the workplace along with the approaches, beliefs, values and attitudes of the individuals of an organization. A wider range of human competence is not only the kind of competence that are relevant to productive work in the economic sector, but also those that human beings need to protect and improve people's health, to deep population growth within reasonable limits, to sustain and develop cultural traditions and identities, to enjoy recreational activities, to put nutritional resources to the best possible use, to preserve a less hazardous and endangered environment, and to assume and play an active role as a citizen. All these competence constitute the society's human resource. The possession of these competencies by an individual to the maximum is possible only through education.

In its broadest meaning education is any process by which an individual gains knowledge or insight, or develops attitudes or skills. Such education can be

- Formal, i.e. acquired through organized study or institution, Or
- Informal, i.e. arise form day-to-day experiences or through relatively unplanned or undirected contacts with communication media.

The function of education is both social and individual. Its social function is to help each individual become a more effective member of society by passing along to him the collective experience of the past and the present. Its individual function is to enable him to lead a more satisfying and productive life by preparing him to handle new experience successfully.

Education takes an important place as the dominant human resource factor. Education is an essential foundation for human resource development. In addition to literacy and numeric skills, basic education for human resource development, involves the inculcation of attitudes and abilities that will promote both a demand for, and the capacity to undertake, further human resource development. Literacy and numeracy and at least a rudimentary understanding of scientific principles and methods are essential pre-conditions for a productive and adaptive population that can utilize and adjust rapidly to new technologies and other exogenous changes. Efforts should therefore be intensified to provide universal basic education. In particular, governments should ensure that basic education is extended to disadvantaged population groups.

Education is also considered to be a form of investment in human capital, which provides workers with knowledge and skills which raise their productivity in employment, and therefore increases future levels of output and national income. Human capital theory postulates that expenditure on education is a form of investment-an investment in human beings. Like investment in any form, investment in human beings gives returns. This return is reflected in the earnings if the educated. This theory postulates that schooling enhances skill and dexterity of individuals which in turn enhances the productivity of the workers. Workers are paid as per their contribution to the total national product. In other words, wages are paid according to the marginal productivity theory of distribution. Hence educated earn more than their less educated counterparts.

Hence education as a form of investment in human capital is analogous to investment in physical capital. Rate of return studies show that:

- Investment in education is profitable
- Private rates of return are higher than social rates of return for any given level of education
- Rates of returns tend to be highest in primary education

World Conference on 'Education for All', gives the Consequences of investments in basic education. According to it, Primary education is known to,

- improve productivity of factory workers.
- help people in the field by providing necessary skills for self-employment and entrepreneurship
- help people to earn higher incomes through informed consumption choices and improved household management
- to contribute to increase in farmer productivity through adoption of technology, use of credit, information and marketing systems
- lead to higher earnings by workers and entrepreneurs
- yield higher rates of both private and social returns than other levels of schooling

In addition,

- increase in literacy was found to contribute to increase in investment and in output per worker
- it was also correlated with increased life expectancy and reduced infant and maternal mortality
- overall differences in patterns of educational investment at national level were found in explaining national rates of economic growth and other indicators of development
- the possession of knowledge and reasoning ability is increasingly defining the individuals and national efficacy. To be deprived of basic education is to be deprived of the essential tools of modern living
- with increased global interdependence education becomes an important tool to reduce disparities and build common cultural understanding within and between nations
- effective education is a unique means to promote participation of individuals in local communities an in the global society

- marginalized populations depend on their knowledge and problem solving skills to deal with the hardships created by war-civil strife and crime as well as discrimination
- increased level of basic learning helps alleviate conditions of disadvantage and thus contribute to reduction of social disparities
- marginalized populations need basic education to prepare them for effective migration social and occupational mobility, access to new information and markets and adaptation to new environment
- increased knowledge helps to inform the individual of the real costs of environment damage and to promote ecologically sound development and land replenishment

Higher education too is a dominant factor in contributing to Human resource. To compete in global markets and create new activities and services developing countries must give emphasis on higher education, since the knowledge and skills required to perform different activities are provided at this level. Contributions of higher education to the nation's human resource development take many forms namely,

1. training of middle and higher level professional, technical and managerial staff
2. creation of new knowledge through research and scientific study
3. training and dissemination
4. forging a cultural identity
5. fostering democratic process by encouraging independent ideas and informed opinions

Education is functionally related to the level of development which a country has achieved or aspires to achieve. Education makes people more productive, by giving them knowledge and skills that improve their work performance and enable them to achieve higher levels of output than uneducated people.

The knowledge and skills required for a developing economy is provided by higher education. The developing countries are proliferating the institutes of higher education and enrolments are also increasing.

The interdependence between educational development and the over-all socio-economic development of a country calls for an analysis of the resource potential in natural, physical and human categories. The exploitation of natural resources depends on the development of human resources and vice-versa. Education plays a significant role in developing human resources. Therefore there is a need to plan education to develop human resources. Education has to be planned in such a way as to develop the human resource potential in order to respond to the needs of the social and economic development of the country, while considering the expectations and attitudes of the people.

SUMMARY

Human resource development consists of three essential Cs, viz., competencies, commitment and culture. HRD needs to be studied in the context of its societal culture and values, since the culture can have a lasting effect on human resource development. A strong culture is a powerful lever for guiding behavior. It helps people to do their jobs better. An effective culture is a system of informal rules that spell out how we are to behave most of the time. It enables people to feel better about what they do, sop they are most likely to work harder. At its core, culture encompasses a set of fundamental values that distinguishes one group from another and these values can act as a strong determinant of managerial ideology that consequently affects both HR practice and performance.

Performance review is a formal exercise in which an organization makes an evaluation of its employees, in terms of contributions made towards achieving organizational objectives and/or their personal strengths and weaknesses, and in terms of attributes and behaviors demonstrated for meeting whatever objectives the organization may consider relevant.

Performance Counseling refers to the help provided by a superior to his subordinate in objectively analyzing their performance. It focuses on the analysis of performance and identification of training and developing needs to bring about further improvement. Its main purpose is employee development. It aims at helping the employee by providing a supportive and empathetic atmosphere in which the employee feels encouraged to discuss his aspirations, tensions, conflicts, concerns and problems. The term, 'Performance counseling' has been replaced by the term, 'Performance Review Discussion (PRD)' in recent times. The counseling process has three phases:

- Rapport building
- Exploration
- Action Planning

Job enrichment is an attempt to *motivate* employees by giving them the opportunity to use the range of their abilities. It is an idea that was developed by the American *psychologist Frederick Herzberg* in the 1950s. Job Enrichment is the addition to a job of tasks that increase the amount of employee control or responsibility. It is a vertical expansion of the job as opposed to the horizontal expansion of a job, which is called job enlargement. Job enrichment is used to make work more challenging and rewarding for employees to make it easier to keep them.

Quality of Working Life is a term that had been used to describe the broader *job*-related experience an individual has. Quality of life and Quality of work are closely interrelated. Quality of Working Life refers to the "degree to which work provides an opportunity for an individual to satisfy a wide variety of personal needs from the need to survive with some security to the need to interact with others, to have a sense of personal usefulness, to be recognized for achievement, and to have an opportunity to improve one's skills and knowledge'.

This linkage between HRD variables will lead to good HRD practices that would help in building competencies and commitment of employees. A wider range of human competence is not only the kind of competence that are relevant to productive work in the economic sector, but also those that human beings need to protect and improve people's health, to deep population growth within reasonable limits, to sustain and develop cultural traditions and identities, to enjoy recreational activities, to put nutritional resources to the best possible use, to preserve a less hazardous and endangered environment, and to assume and play an active role as a citizen. All these competence constitute the society's human resource. The possession of these competencies by an individual to the maximum is possible only through education. Education takes an important place as the dominant human resource factor. Education is an essential foundation for human resource development. In addition to literacy and numeric skills, basic education for human resource development, involves the inculcation of attitudes and abilities that will promote both a demand for, and the capacity to undertake, further human resource development.

BIBLIOGRAPHY

Alan Cranston (1992) - Human Resources Division - United States, Washington, D.C.

AHRD Conference- (2002) - Approaches to Research in HRD— U.S. Department of Education. U.S.A.

AHRD conference (2001) - Role of HRD in women's career development - Department of Education, U.S.A

Argyris, C. Schori. D.A. (1978) - Organisational learning - Addison-Wesley Publishing Company, U.S.A

Ashwatappa - "Human Resource Management", Tata McGraw Publications.

Donald bforwhat (2007) - Changing Nature of Human Resource Management-U.S.A

Eisenhardt, Kathleen, M. Eisenhard (1989) - Building theories from case study research - U.S.A

Elliot Chocron, Matthew Steigerwald (2003) - Role of functional and cross-functional planning in managing the enterprise

Fisher schoenfeldt Shaw – "Human Resource Management", HoughtonMifflin publishers, U.S.A.

Gary Desler – "Human Resource management" - Pearson publications.

John bratton, Jeffrey Gold (2003)- Human Resource Management-U.S.A.

Kenneth Bartlett, Karen Johnson, and Ingrid E. Schneider (2006) - A Comparative Study of Strategic HRD Approaches, U.S.A.

Madhava Rao- (2008) – Human Resource Development, Training & Skill Development, Ministry of HRD, India.

Milkovich, G. T., and Newman, J. M. (2005). Compensation [Eighth Edition]. Tata McGraw-Hill Publishing Company Limited.

Maslow, A. H. (1943). A theory of human motivation. *Psychological Review, 50*, 370-396

Mamoria, Gaonkar - "Personnel Management".

Nair, Latha Nair - "Personnel Management and Industrial Relations".

Pilar Jerez Go mez and Jose J. Ce´spedes Lorente-(2003) - Training practices and organizational learning capability relationship and implications, Spain.

Pareek U., Rao T.V. (1986) - "Designing and managing Human Resources systems, Oxford IBH.

Rao,T.V. (1984) Performance appraisal - Theory and Practice AIMA Vikas series, New Delhi.

Rao, T.V, Verma K.K., Anil, K. Khandelwad. E. Abeaham S.J. (1997) - "Alternative approaches and HRD"- Rawat publications, New Delhi.

Rao VSP, Narayana "Organisational Theory and Behaviour", Konark Publishers, New Delhi.

Rakesh Chopra - "Management of Human Resources".

Shaveta Arya (2008) - Leadership challenges among HR professionals - Exploratory study Bombay.

Sharma, R.K., Shashi K. Gupta (2000) "Business Management", Kalyani Publishers, New Delhi.

Schein, A. (1984) - "Career development: Issues for organizations", McGraw Hill Co.

Subba Rao - "Essentials of Human Resource Management and Industrial Relation", Himalaya Publishing House, New Delhi.

Subba Rao - "Personal and Human Resource Management", Himalaya Publishing House, New Delhi.

Venkataratanam, Srinivastava (1997) - "Personnel Management and Human Resources", McGraw Hill Co.

Werner, Desimone (2006) - Evaluating HRD programs - U.S.A

www.emeraldinsight.com

www.sagepub.com

www.hrd.com

—00—